BADASS
BRAIDS

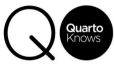

Brimming with creative inspiration, how-to projects, and useful information to enrich your everyday life, Quarto Knows is a favorite destination for those pursuing their interests and passions. Visit our site and dig deeper with our books into your area of interest: Quarto Creates, Quarto Cooks, Quarto Homes, Quarto Lives, Quarto Drives, Quarto Explores, Quarto Gifts, or Quarto Kids.

Text and photographs on pages 42, 47, 88, 104, 134, 140, 150, 156 © 2018 by Shannon Burns

First published in 2018 by Race Point, an imprint of The Quarto Group,
142 West 36th Street, 4th Floor, New York, NY 10018, USA
T (212) 779-4972 **F** (212) 779-6058 **www.QuartoKnows.com**

Race Point titles are also available at discount for retail, wholesale, promotional, and bulk purchase. For details, contact the Special Sales Manager by email at specialsales@quarto.com or by mail at The Quarto Group, Attn: Special Sales Manager, 401 Second Avenue North, Suite 310, Minneapolis, MN 55401, USA.

10 9 8 7 6 5 4 3 2 1

ISBN: 978-1-63106-438-8

Editorial Director: Jeannine Dillon
Creative Director: Merideth Harte
Managing Editor: Erin Canning
Project Editor: Melanie Madden
Photography: Frank Horn
Illustration: Fortuna Todisco
Cover Design: Merideth Harte
Interior Design: Melissa Gerber
Illustrations on pages 15–19 © Shutterstock

Printed in China

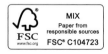

Badass Braids

FROM VIKINGS TO GAME OF THRONES

45 MAVERICK BRAIDS, BUNS, AND TWISTS FOR SCI-FI AND FANTASY FANATICS

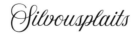

SHANNON BURNS

CREATOR AND HOST OF THE
POPULAR YOUTUBE CHANNEL
Silvousplaits

Race Point
PUBLISHING

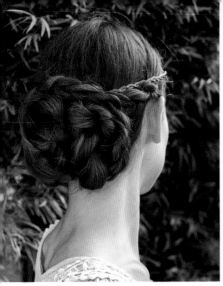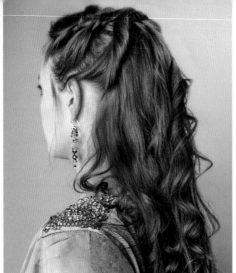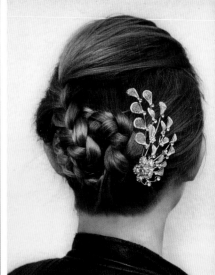

Contents

INTRODUCTION 7

STYLING TOOLS & TRICKS 9

BASIC BRAIDS 15

CHAPTER 1: ANCIENT ADVERSARIES 21

Atia of the Julii, Inspired by *Rome* 23

Gannicus, Inspired by
Spartacus: War of the Damned 27

Gorgo Queen of Sparta, Inspired by *300* 29

Lucretia, Inspired by
Spartacus: Blood and Sand 33

CHAPTER 2: VIKING WARRIORS 37

Uhtred of Bebbanburg,
Inspired by *The Last Kingdom* 39

Kwenthrith, Queen of Mercia Inspired by
Vikings 43

Ragnar Lothbrok, Inspired by *Vikings* 45

Torvi, Inspired by *Vikings* 49

Lagertha, Inspired by *Vikings* 53

CHAPTER 3: RENAISSANCE ROYALS 57

Anne Boleyn, Inspired by *The Tudors* 59

Mary Queen of Scots, Inspired by *Reign* 61

Lucrezia Borgia, Inspired by *The Borgias* 65

Elizabeth of York, Inspired by
The White Princess 69

CHAPTER 4: ROMANTIC RENEGADES 73

Vanessa Ives, Inspired by *Penny Dreadful* 75

Charles Vane, Inspired by *Black Sails* 79

Jenny Murray, Inspired by *Outlander* 81

Max, Inspired by *Black Sails* 85

Lizzy Bennet, Inspired by
Pride and Prejudice 89

CHAPTER 5: FIERCE FANTASY 93

Emma Swan, Inspired by
Once Upon a Time 95

Margaery Tyrell, Inspired by
Game of Thrones 99

Diana Prince, Inspired by
Wonder Woman 101

Legolas, Inspired by
The Lord of the Rings 105

Morgana Pendragon, Inspired by *Merlin* 107

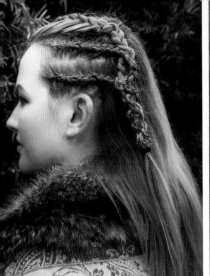 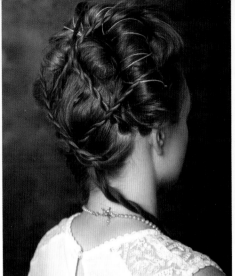 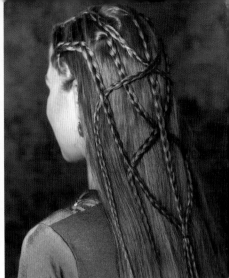

Daenerys Targaryen, Inspired by
    Game of Thrones......................................111
Éowyn, Inspired by
    The Lord of the Rings: The Two Towers 115
Tauriel, Inspired by *The Hobbit*.................117
Cersei Lannister, Inspired by
    Game of Thrones......................................121
Eretria, Inspired by
    The Shannara Chronicles 125
Sansa Stark, Inspired by
    Game of Thrones......................................129

CHAPTER 6: SCI-FI HEROINES **133**
Rey, Inspired by
    Star Wars: The Force Awakens..................135
Gamora, Inspired by
    Guardians of the Galaxy...........................137
Cressida, Inspired by
    The Hunger Games: Mockingjay..............141
Leia Organa, Inspired by
    Star Wars: The Empire Strikes Back..........145
Maeve Millay, Inspired by *Westworld* 147

Padmé Amidala, Inspired by
    Star Wars: Revenge of the Sith 151
Katniss Everdeen, Inspired by
    The Hunger Games: Mockingjay..............153
Octavia Blake, Inspired by *The 100*...........157
Deanna Troi, Inspired by
    Star Trek: The Next Generation 161

CHAPTER 7: ANIMATED ADVENTURISTS... 165
Usagi Tsukino, Inspired by *Sailor Moon*.....167
Zelda, Inspired by
    The Legend of Zelda: Twilight Princess.....169
Katara, Inspired by
    Avatar: The Last Airbender 173
Evie Frye, Inspired by *Assassin's Creed*.........177
Astrid Hofferson, Inspired by
    How to Train Your Dragon 2 179
Lunafreya Nox Fleuret, Inspired by
    Final Fantasy...183
Aloy, Inspired by *Horizon Zero Dawn*........187

ACKNOWLEDGMENTS **191**

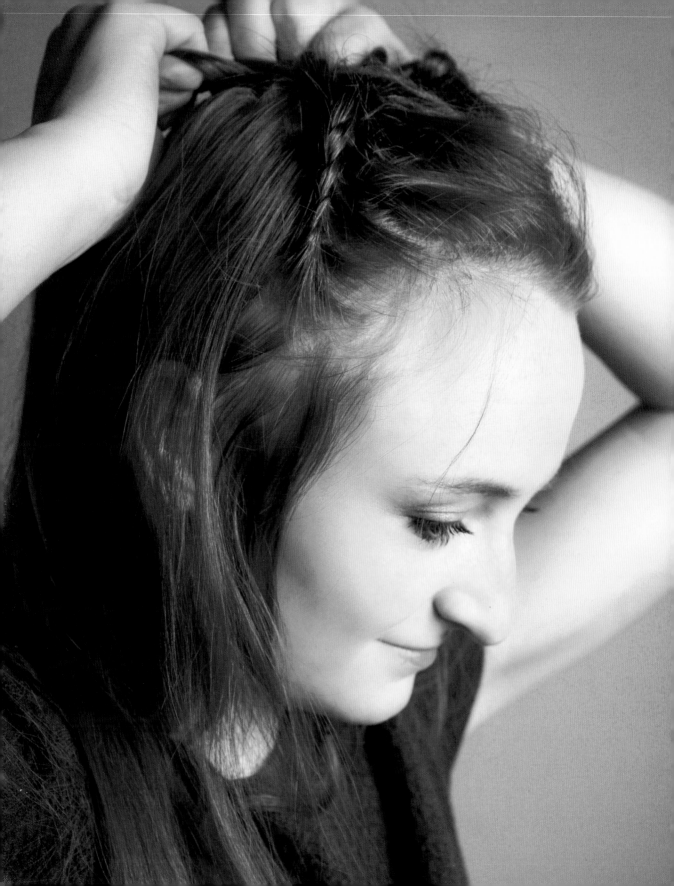

{ Introduction }

*Welcome to Badass Braids, your ultimate guide
to fantasy and sci-fi hairstyling!*

From the gladiator ring to the courts of Renaissance queens, from the lands of Middle-earth to a galaxy far, far away, the creativity displayed by today's costume dramas—in film and television—is simply amazing. Their strong characters and richly crafted worlds have inspired massive followings, and lots of people want to bring a bit of otherworldliness into their daily lives. One simple and powerful way to do so is to duplicate the characters' hairstyles, and that's my goal with this book: to teach you how to recreate the best hairstyles from your favorite shows and movies on yourself and others.

I have always loved hairstyling because the possibilities are endless and it gives you so much confidence. At the same time, I'm a big nerd. For the last several years I have studied and replicated the hairstyles in my favorite TV shows and

movies, including *Game of Thrones*, *Outlander*, *Lord of the Rings*, and *The Hunger Games*. Originally I began doing it just for my own amusement, but when I created my Silvousplaits YouTube channel and started posting tutorials for all to see, I discovered how much fun it was to share my passion for hairstyling with others.

This book is the culmination of that process, offering 45 of my favorite hairstyles from several popular and geeky movies, shows, and video games—all presented with the DIY stylist in mind. The styles are arranged by genre into separate chapters, each of which features hairstyles for a variety of hair lengths, textures, and skill levels. Step-by-step instructions and illustrations will teach you how to achieve these looks on yourself, and behind-the-scenes information from show stylists will shed light on how the hairstyles were developed, including how they evolve with the character and which historical techniques and tools they incorporate. Fantasy and sci-fi hairstyling is not your everyday "ponytail and go" sort of approach to hair, so the book begins with an introduction to the styling tools you'll need and simple instructions for the types of braids used to achieve these looks. Read this section first. Once you master the fundamentals, you will be ready to create some awesome hairstyles!

My philosophy is that hairstyling is an art form you can wear, enabling you to transform yourself and even be a whole new person for a day. By following the instructions in this book, you'll be able to elevate your personal style and channel the essence of some of the most badass heroes and heroines from fiction and history.

Have fun!

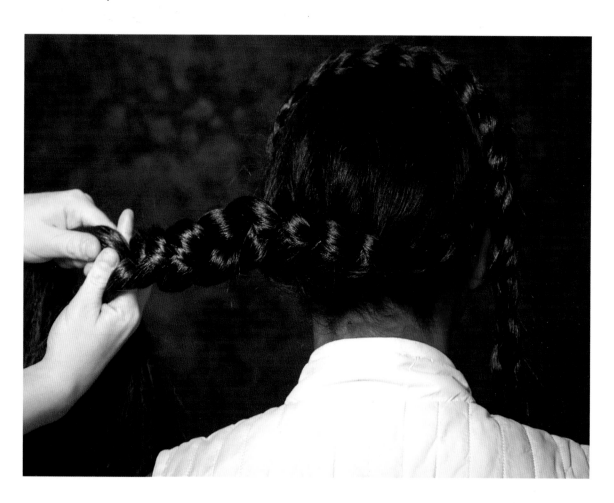

{ Styling Tools & Tricks }

Here are the basic materials you will need to create the styles in this book. Many of them will work for all hair types, but depending on the thickness and length of your hair, you may need to rely more on certain materials and products.

Hairbrushes & Combs

The most basic hairstyling tools. If you have a head of hair, you likely own a brush or comb. Combs are best for smoothing out hair and for precision work, but they tend to make tangles worse by pushing them together into a tight knot. Brushes, on the other hand, are best for detangling. The softer the bristles, the gentler the brush will be, but beware: this also means the hair will take longer to detangle. Boar bristle brushes are also popular, as the natural fibers redistribute scalp oils to make your hair shinier.

Hair Tip

My favorite everyday brush is called the Tangle Teezer, which has an ergonomic hold and flexible bristles that don't rip through tangles.

Hair Clips

Many of the styles in this book require you to section your hair in various ways. To hold these sections separate while you work, you'll need some hair clips. My favorite are duck-bill clips, because they're easy to insert. You can also use claw clips for added grip.

Rattail Comb

Rattail combs, or teasing combs, have a dual purpose: the thin, tightly packed teeth enable you to tease hair effectively, while the pointed end of the comb can be used as a sectioning tool. To make nice and straight sections in your hair, simply place the pointed end against your scalp and draw a line where you want the section to be.

Hair Elastics

Hair elastics come in many sizes and colors, as well as a variety of materials, such as rubber or fabric. It's useful to have a variety of sizes, colors, and materials on hand. Small and clear elastics are good for the ends of braids, particularly when you want to hide the braid end underneath a bun. Large, soft-surfaced hair elastics are better for making ponytails with big sections of hair, since these elastics are easier to remove without snagging the hair elastics. For added comfort, elastic ribbon ties are also available, as well as a telephone-cord-like tie called Invisibobble, which leaves no ponytail crease!

Hair Pins

Bobby pins are really useful for getting hair to stay in whatever position you want it. When you make buns, twists, and generally any shape that involves defying gravity, bobby pins will usually be involved. You can use these to attach one section of hair to another place on the head, and for extra hold, you can cross two bobby pins in an X shape. Note that the flat top of the bobby pin should face outward, allowing the wavy part to scoop up hair as you slide it along your scalp. Generally, you want to hide your bobby pins for a nice clean look, so slide them underneath braids and buns.

Some related tools include spin pins and U-shaped hair pins. Spin pins are modern corkscrew-like inventions that stay positioned better—especially in thick hair—when they are rotated into a bun or other updo. U-shaped hair pins have been around much longer and can hold bigger sections of hair than the smaller bobby pins. Once you master bobby pins, you can practice using these.

Topsy Tail

A topsy tail is a simple plastic device that works like a giant needle and is used to flip ponytails inside out or to weave one section of hair through another. To use it, simply thread a section of hair through the large hole in the topsy tail, then use the pointed end to push the topsy tail through whatever hair you want to weave through (e.g., under a hair elastic or through the strands of another braid). When you pull the topsy tail out the other side, the section of hair you threaded through the hole comes with it. Topsy tails can be bought online very cheaply.

Hair Beads

Hair beads have been used for millennia all around the world, and they are incorporated into many styles on the screen today. You can buy dedicated hair beads that are high quality and artistic, but in a pinch, you can also use any sort of crafting bead.

There are many ways to use hair beads, but I generally use them as decoration on top of hair elastics that are already holding twists and braids together. Slide the bead onto the hair either by wetting the hair ends and poking them through the bead hole, or by using a loop of thread to pull the hair through the hole, like a makeshift topsy tail. To keep the bead in place, slide it up high enough so that it is very tight on the hair, or slide it on top of a small hair elastic, which provides enough friction to hold it in place.

Hair Extensions

For much of history, it's been fashionable to have long, voluminous hair, and today is no different. This is why many hairstyles in television and film require actors to wear extensions, which add length and thickness. Extensions are exceptionally useful if your hair is on the fine or thin side and you're going for a screen-accurate look.

Most extensions are either clip-in or free hanging. Clip-in extensions can be secured to the roots of your own hair or to hair inserts. Free-hanging extensions can be twisted or braided into separate hair pieces and then pinned to your head. Many retail companies sell hair extensions, so search online to find a set that has good reviews and fits your budget. It's best to buy extensions that are as close a match to your own hair color as possible. If you can't find your color—shout-out to my fellow redheads, it's a struggle—buy blonde extensions and then ask a stylist to color them for you.

Hair Tip

If you're buying your own extensions, I recommend getting real hair if you can afford it. (Fake hair is often noticeably different in texture when mixed in with your own hair.)

Hair Inserts

Hair inserts come in a wide variety of sizes and are meant to help give volume to updos, so you don't have to use any of your own limited hair to create the basic hairstyle structure. Many people are familiar with the foam rings known as hair donuts. You can also get roll shapes (either by buying a hair roll or by cutting a hair donut in half), small hair bumps for just a little added volume, and bigger beehive inserts that are shaped like a ball. These accessories are available all over the internet from many retailers, so just use these terms as keywords to search!

Hair Tip

Don't have any hair inserts? You can make your own! Simply ball up some cheap hair extensions, manipulate them into the shape you want, and then secure them all together with a hairnet. You can even use hair collected from your hairbrush (which is what women did historically).

Sprays & Serums

There are probably a million and a half different styling products out there, but most fall into a few categories based on their function. In our case, the most useful products are hairsprays and texture sprays. Hairspray holds hair in whatever position you need but is sticky until it dries. You can use it before curling your hair so the shape holds better or to keep a look in place at the end of styling. Texture sprays go on dry, and they give your hair more grip, which is helpful when making loose braids or fluffed-out twists that are otherwise prone to falling out. Texture sprays are a major help for people with slippery hair!

Other products you'll want to have on hand are a heat protectant (in case you're using heat tools), as well as shine spray and/or pomade. Shine sprays are usually used before styling to make frizzy hair more manageable, but they can also go on at the end as a finishing touch. Pomades are helpful for smoothing down sections of hair before braiding or after the style is finished to create a sleek look. Don't be afraid to be creative and experiment with the products you try and at what point in the styling pipeline you use them!

Heat Tools

Heat tools are really useful whenever you want to change your hair's basic shape—either by curling, crimping, or straightening. For curling, you can use a curling iron (which has a metal clamp to keep your hair attached to the iron), a curling wand (no metal clamp), or hot rollers that you heat up separately and then place in your hair. If you wrap smaller sections of hair around a curling tool and keep them there for a longer period of time, the curl will last longer, but beware: more heat equals more hair damage.

Crimping irons are great for putting micro texture in your hair, which improves its grip and volume. For those of you with fine or thin hair who don't want to use extensions, the added volume that crimping provides is quite astounding!

For those with naturally textured hair who want a smoother look, a straightening iron or straightening brush makes the hair straighter until your next wash. Take one small, flat section of hair at a time, and slowly run the straightening tool down the length. You may need to do a couple of passes to achieve the desired look.

Hair Tip

Rub pomade on your hands before you start braiding to limit "braid shred" (all those little hairs that stick out of finished braids).

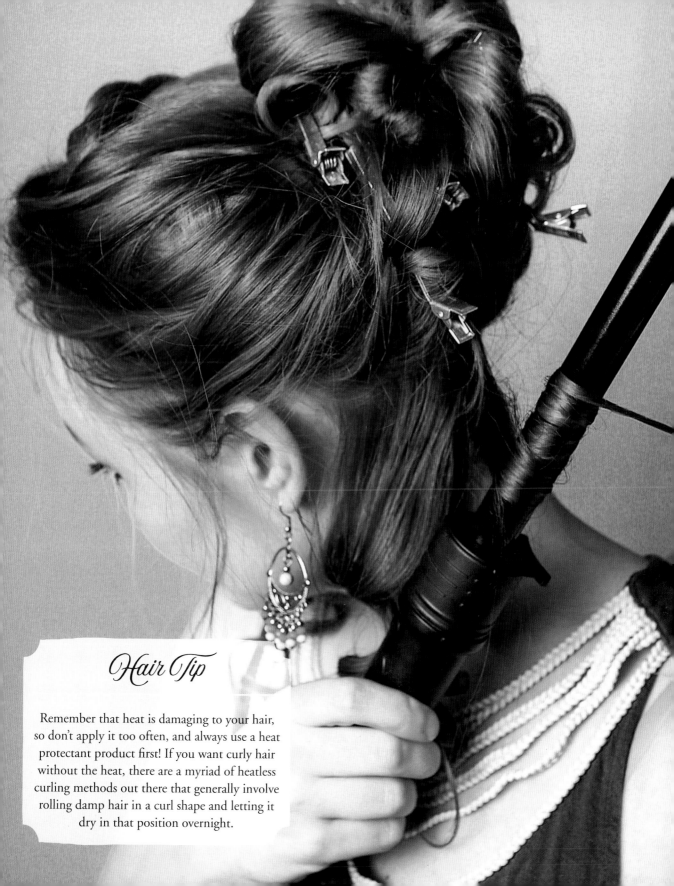

Hair Tip

Remember that heat is damaging to your hair, so don't apply it too often, and always use a heat protectant product first! If you want curly hair without the heat, there are a myriad of heatless curling methods out there that generally involve rolling damp hair in a curl shape and letting it dry in that position overnight.

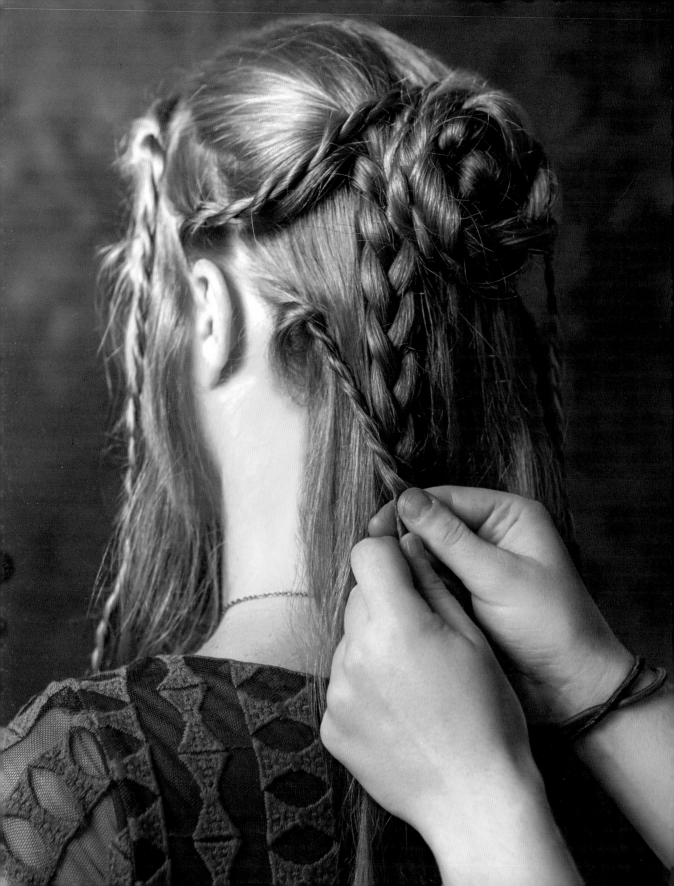

{ BASIC BRAIDS }

This book involves a lot of braiding, so you'll need to learn a few basic types of braids in order to complete these hairstyles. The easier braids shouldn't take you very long to master. The more complex ones will require some practice to remember which strands go where, in what order, and how to most effectively position the strands in your fingers.

English Braid

The English braid is just the fancy name for a normal three-strand braid. After splitting your hair into three strands, weave one of the outer strands over the middle one, so the two switch places. Then weave the outer strand on the opposite side over the middle one, so it becomes the new middle strand. Continue this alternating pattern to the ends of your hair.

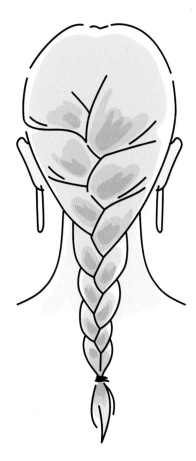

French Braid

The French braid uses the same alternating pattern as the English braid, where you take turns weaving the outer strands over the middle one. The big difference is that before each outer strand is woven over the middle, more hair is added to the strand, making it bigger.

Dutch Braid

Like the French braid, the Dutch braid is another three-strand braid that involves adding in new hair to each outer strand before weaving. The difference is that the outer strands are woven under the middle strand instead of over, making the braid look as if it's sitting on top of your head.

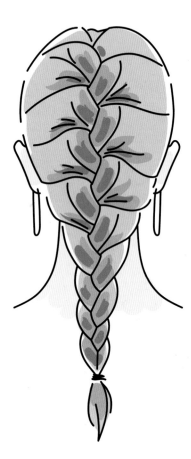
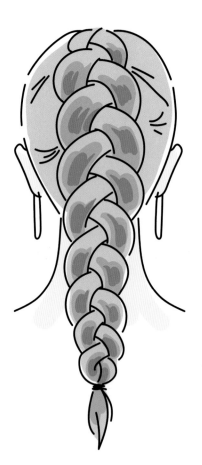

Lace Braid

For a lace braid, new hair is added only on one side of the braid, meaning that if new hair is added to the left-hand strand, no new hair is added to the right-hand strand. Lace braids can be done in either a French variation (outer strands weaving over the middle) or a Dutch variation (outer strands weaving under the middle).

Waterfall Braid

A waterfall braid is basically the opposite of a lace braid, in that before you weave each outer strand over the middle, you remove some hair from the strand and let that hair fall away. You'll also need to add hair to waterfall braids if you don't want the braid to run out of hair. Two ways of doing so involve (1) adding in hair to strands on one side of the braid and removing hair from strands on the other side, and (2) removing hair and then adding in new hair to each of the outer strands in turn.

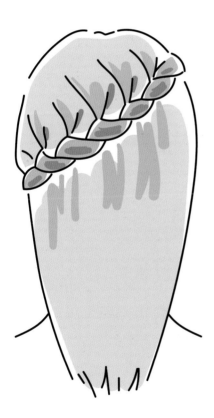

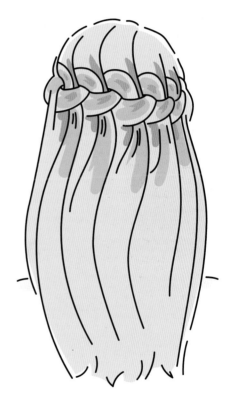

Rope Braid

Rope braids involve just two strands of hair. To get them to hold together, you must first twist the individual strands in one direction, and then twist them around each other in the opposite direction. I find it easiest to make rope braids by twisting one strand individually a couple of times, twisting the two strands together in the opposite direction 180 degrees, twisting the other strand individually a couple of times, doing another half twist with the two strands, and so on. You can do French and lace versions of the rope braid, too—just add new hair to both strands (French) or only to one strand (lace) every time you twist them together.

Fishtail Braid

To begin this braid, divide your hair in half. Break off a little bit of hair from the outside of one half, bring it over, and add it to the inside of the other half of hair. Then break off some hair from the outside of the other half and add it to the inside of the first half. Repeat this alternating pattern for the length of the braid. French or lace variations of the fishtail braid can be done as well, and the Dutch fishtail involves weaving the little bits of hair from the outside underneath the braid instead of over it.

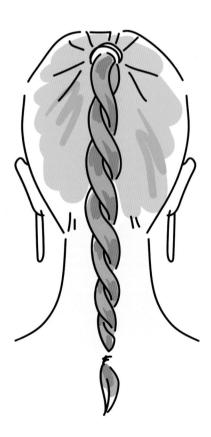

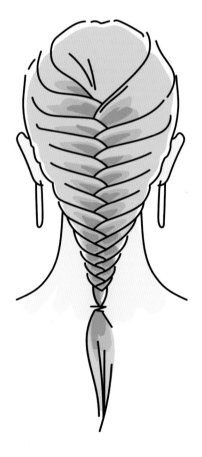

Knot Braid

When knot braiding, just think macramé—making knots with your hair! It might sound scary at first, but remember that hair is quite elastic. (If you tie sections of hair into a knot, it's pretty easy to loosen them again.) There are many different kinds of knot braids, but the kind used in this book is the simplest version, in which you take one strand of hair and tie it into a square knot around another strand. Tighten this knot, and repeat.

Four- & Five-Strand Braids

There are a few different types of four- and five-strand braids. In this book we'll be using the traverse variation, in which one outer strand "traverses" its way through the other strands and then ends up as the outer strand on the other side of the braid. To start, separate your hair into four or five strands. Weave the outermost strand on one side of the braid over the next strand, under the following strand, over the one after that, and so on until it is on the opposite side of the braid. Go back to the first side of the braid again, take the new outermost strand, and weave it over, under, and over the other strands. Repeat this for the entire length of the braid.

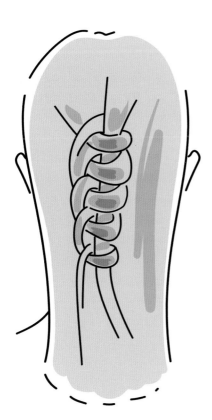

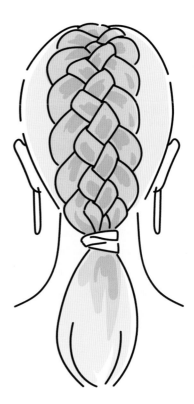

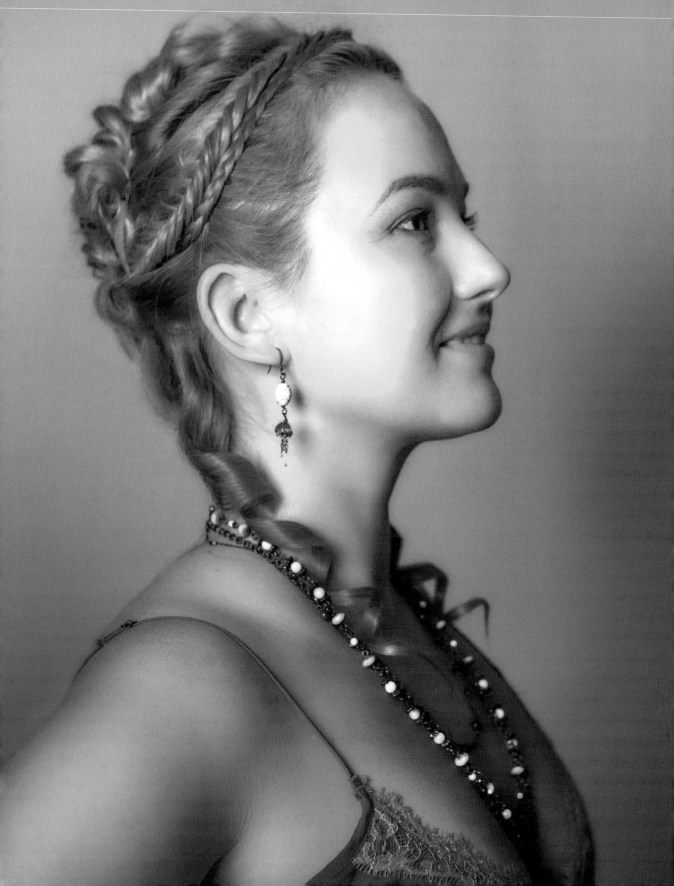

CHAPTER 1

Ancient Adversaries

How one's hair was styled was an important indication of status in Ancient Rome and Greece. In this chapter we will be recreating the hairstyles of characters from the historical drama series *Rome* and *Spartacus*, as well as the Frank Miller–inspired film *300*. In the latter we find **Gorgo, Queen of Sparta**, helping to rally 300 Spartans into taking arms against the ruthless Persian king Xerxes and his army of 300,000 in 478 BCE. *Rome*, which aired on HBO from 2005 to 2007, centers on the exciting period of first-century BCE Roman history as the republic transformed into a vast empire. Among the power players in this Emmy Award–winning drama is Julius Caesar's niece **Atia of the Julii**, a conniving noblewoman who competes with Cleopatra for the affections of Mark Antony. *Spartacus*, which aired on Starz between 2010 and 2013, is based on the story of the historical Thracian gladiator who led slaves in a massive uprising against their Roman captors from 73 to 71 BCE. One of Spartacus's generals in the rebellion is the Celtic ex-gladiator **Gannicus**. On the other side of the conflict is **Lucretia**, a femme fatale like *Rome*'s Atia who carries on an affair with an enslaved Gallic gladiator and murders her political enemies.

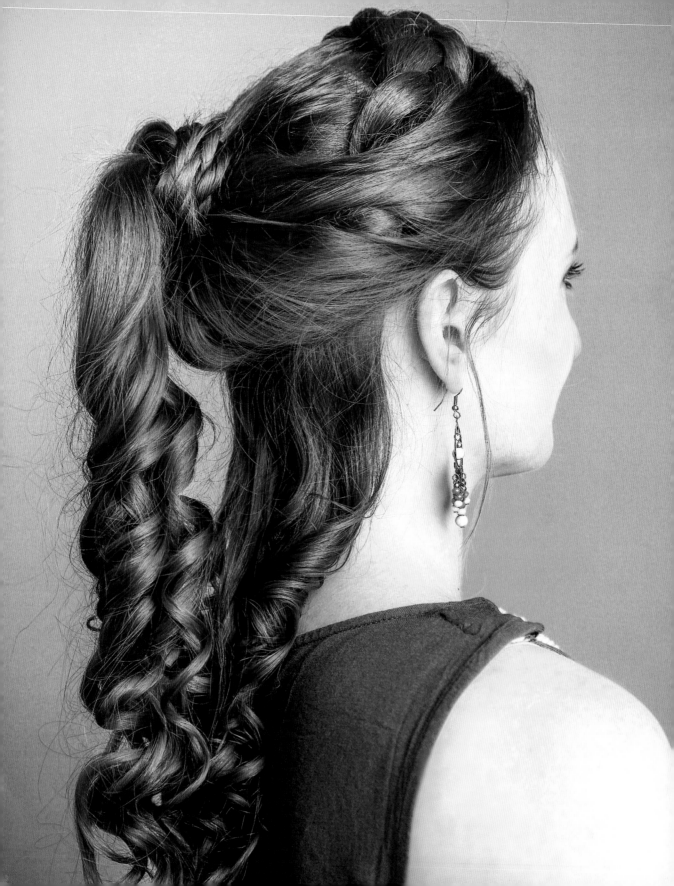

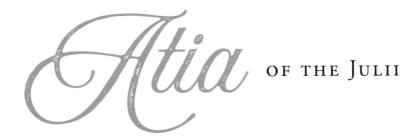

OF THE JULII

Played by English actress Polly Walker, the character of Atia is (very loosely) based on Julius Caesar's actual niece, the pious Atia Balba (85–43 BCE), who became the mother of Rome's first emperor, Augustus. However, interviews with the series creators reveal that Atia of the Julii's character takes more inspiration from the highly educated—and extremely scandalous—Roman noblewoman-poet Clodia Metelli (born ca. 95 BCE). A notorious drinker and gambler, Clodia had numerous extramarital affairs, taking slaves and married men as lovers. Nicknamed Medea of the Palatine by Cicero (in reference to the legendary sorceress who murdered her own children), Clodia was even suspected of poisoning her husband in 59 BCE.

Here, we learn to recreate one of the hairstyles the fictional Atia wears for her ostentatious parties aimed at currying favor with Caesar.

SKILL LEVEL: Easy
TIME: 15 minutes

MATERIALS NEEDED:

18-inch-plus (45 cm) hair extensions

1 large hair elastic

Bobby pins

1 small, clear hair elastic

Curling iron

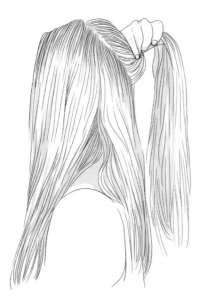

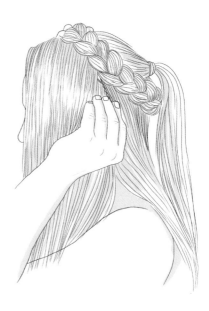

I. Gather up the hair at the crown and tie it into a ponytail.

2. English-braid the hair extension, and then pin it to the head so that it wraps over the top of the head and the ends meet underneath the ponytail.

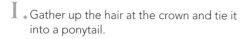

{ **DID YOU KNOW?**

Greek women would often use intricate wraps and netting to secure their hair up on their heads, and Roman women had specially trained slaves called *ornatrices* who spent a great deal of time creating elaborate hair designs.

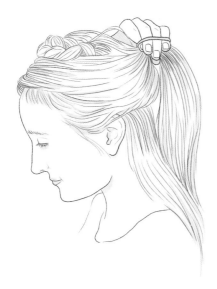

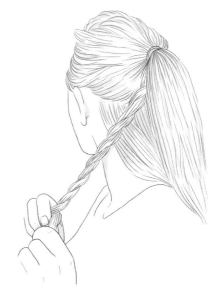

3. Except for a section of hair at the nape of the neck, drape the rest of the hair over the braid so that only the part of braid at the top of the head shows. Join this hair to the ponytail and retie it.

4. Take a 1- to 2-inch (2.5 to 5 cm) section of the ponytail and rope-braid it. Secure the ends with a small, clear elastic.

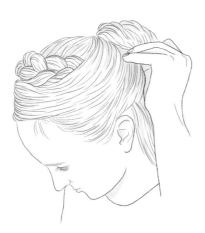

5. Wrap this rope braid around the base of the ponytail, pinning it in place with bobby pins. Then use the curling iron to make ringlets in the ponytail and the hair hanging underneath.

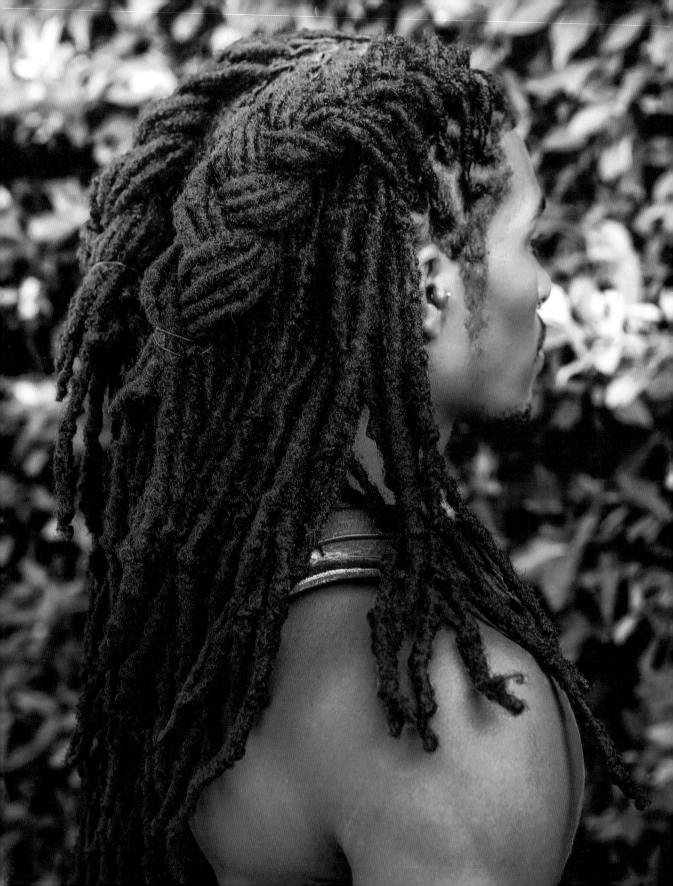

Gannicus

Known as "God of the Arena" and portrayed by the Australian actor Dustin Clare in the *Spartacus* television series, the character of Gannicus is based on a real Celtic slave who helped command the so-called "Gladiator War" against the Roman Republic and met his end in the winter of 71 BCE, near present-day Mount Soprano in southern Italy. By the fourth and final season, *War of the Damned*, Gannicus has become the only gladiator ever to win his freedom through his unparalleled fighting prowess in the arena, and he has decided, in honor of his dear fallen friend Oenomaus, to join Spartacus's rebellion.

SKILL LEVEL: Easy
TIME: 10 minutes

MATERIALS NEEDED:

2 small hair elastics

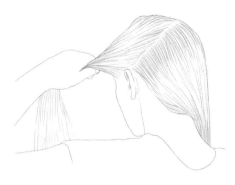

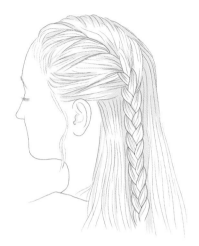

1. Make a center part, and then draw another part on either side of the head, extending from behind the ear up to the crown of the head. These two triangular sections on top of the head will become the French braids.

2. Tie the rest of the hair out of the way at the back of the head. Pick up a small amount of hair at the forehead in one of the two triangular sections. Split this hair into three strands and start French braiding toward the back of the head. When there is no more hair in this first section to add in, English-braid to the ends and secure it with one of the hair elastics.

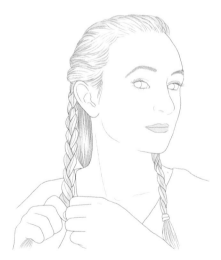

3. Repeat step 2 with the triangular section of hair on the other side. Let down the rest of the hair to finish the look.

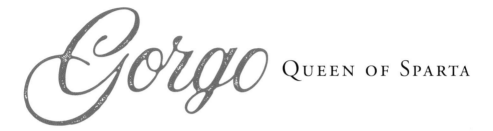

Gorgo Queen of Sparta

Played by the English actress Lena Headey, the character of Gorgo is (somewhat loosely) based on the real-life Queen of Sparta (born ca. 518 to 508 BCE), who was the only known child of the brilliant but reckless Spartan ruler Cleomenes I. She married her father's half-brother, King Leonides I, and assisted him during the Persian invasion of 480 BCE. Gorgo's deeds were recorded by the fifth-century Greek historian Herodotus, who commended her for being both wise and strategic.

Queen Gorgo wears this hairstyle at the beginning of the movie *300* as Leonides departs for the war with Persia.

SKILL LEVEL: Intermediate
TIME: 20 minutes

MATERIALS NEEDED:

7 small, clear hair elastics

Scissors

A decorative string or cord that is at least 8 times the length of the hair

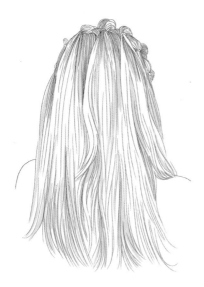

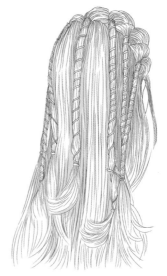

1. Divide the hair on the top of the head into seven equal sections: one in the center, one from each corner of the forehead, and two more on each side of the head. Secure each of these sections with a small, clear elastic.

2. Cut 8 lengths of string or cord that are at least as long as the hair. Thread one end of one strand through the elastic on one of the sections of hair and then twist it around the hair. When there are just a couple of inches of string left, tie it in a knot around the hair to secure it in place. Repeat this step for the remaining six sections of hair, creating seven wrapped sections in total.

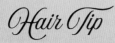

Hair Tip

If you don't have enough hair to make seven twists, make five instead, with just one twist on each side of the head.

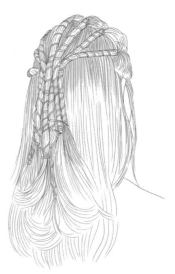

3. Bring all of the twists together at the center of the back of the head. Weave the last length of string around them to hold them together. Knot the string underneath to keep the sections tightly secured together.

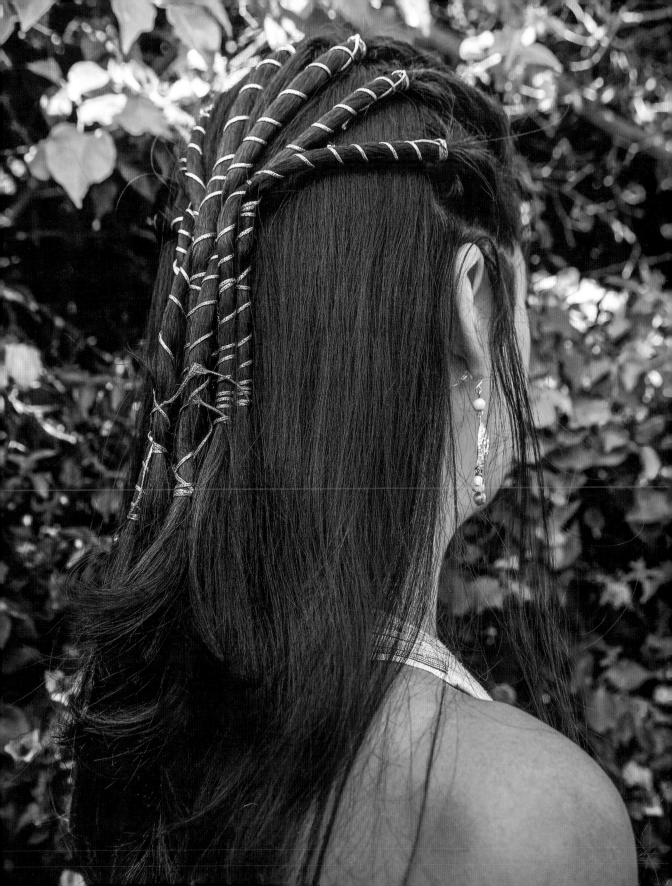

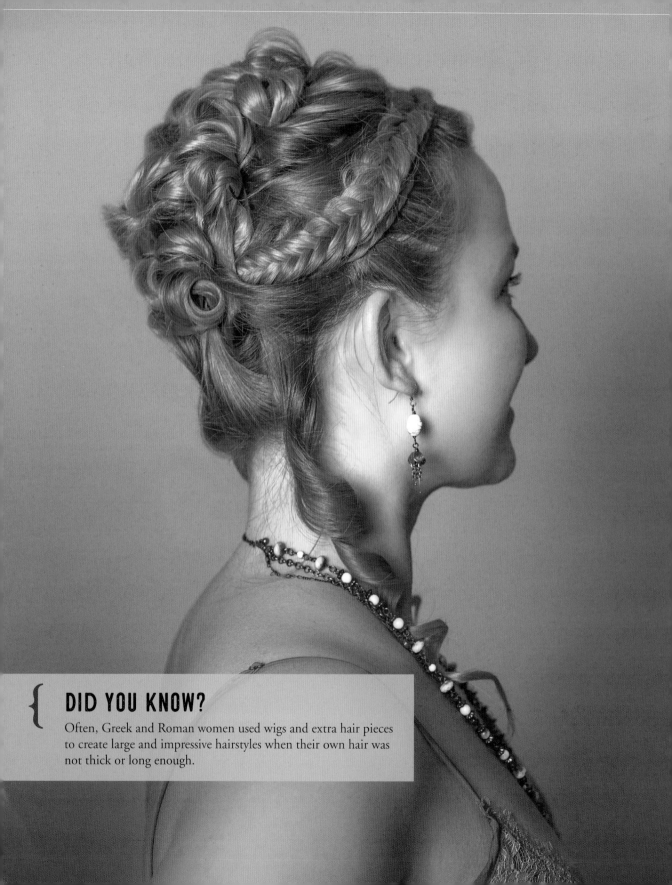

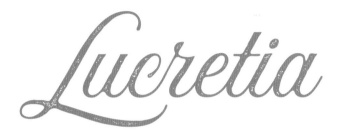

Played by the Kiwi actress Lucy Lawless, Lucretia is as ambitious and ruthless as Batiatus, her husband. Batiatus, who owns the *ludus* in Capua where Spartacus trains to become a gladiator, seeks power and government favor by securing spots for his fighters in prestigious games. Lucretia plays the soft-power game by cultivating important friends, dressing fashionably, and building a reputation of procuring certain "entertainment" for Capua's elite.

This complex and elegant hairstyle can be seen in the fourth episode of *Blood and Sand*, when Lucretia and Batiatus are scheming about how to make more money from the fighting pits.

SKILL LEVEL: Advanced
TIME: 30 minutes

MATERIALS NEEDED:

3 small, clear hair elastics

Hair clips

Bobby pins

Curling iron

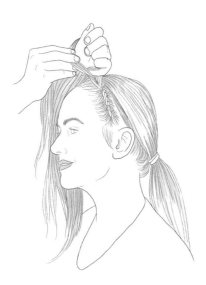

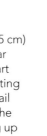

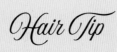

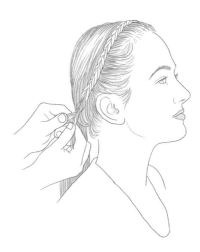

I. Part the hair so there is a 2-inch-wide (5 cm) section along the forehead, running ear to ear. Tilt the head to the side and start braiding this "headband" section, starting from the left side, as a Dutch lace fishtail braid. Form the braid over the top of the head and down the other side, picking up new hair from the headband section you made until there is no more hair to add.

2. Fishtail-braid the rest of this hair to the ends and secure with a small, clear hair elastic.

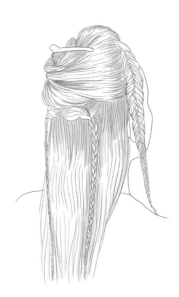

Hair Tip

If your hair is too short to make braids that can wrap around your head, or your hair is too thin to make them look nice, you can use hair extensions to make the braids and then pin these to your head before curling your own hair and making the curl bun.

3. Horizontally divide the rest of the hair in half. Clip the hair above this part out of the way for now. Make two English braids from two small sections of hair at the back of the head, taking these sections from right below the part. Braid to the ends and secure with small hair elastics.

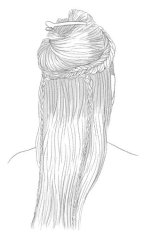

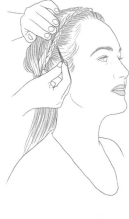

4. Pin the fishtail braid behind the head, along the horizontal part. If it's long enough, drape it back around the head and pin it along the beginning of the fishtail at the front of the head.

5. Drape the leftmost English braid around the left side of the head and along the fishtail braid in front. Pin it in place. Then drape the other English braid around the right side of the head and along the fishtail in front. Make sure to tuck and pin the ends of each braid underneath the other braids to hide the hair elastics from view.

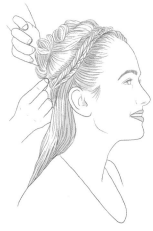

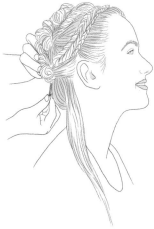

6. Using the curling iron, curl the hair below the braids in sections 1 to 2 inches (2.5 to 5 cm) wide by wrapping the section around the iron and holding for about ten seconds. Unclip the hair above the horizontal part and curl it as well. Then pick up one curl at the top of the head and wrap it tightly around a couple of fingers to form a coil about 1 inch (2.5 cm) in diameter. Pin it to the top of the head. Repeat this step with the rest of the hair above the horizontal part, pinning them close together to create a soft and romantic-looking curly bun at the top back of the head.

7. Pick up a chunk of hair behind the ears now and split it in half. Then coil and pin up the half closest to the ear, clipping the other half out of the way for now. Repeat this step on the other side of the head. Coil and pin up the rest of the hair to finish the curl bun, making sure to cover the braids in the back of the head. Then unclip the two tendrils of hair you left out of the bun and let them hang over the shoulders to finish the look.

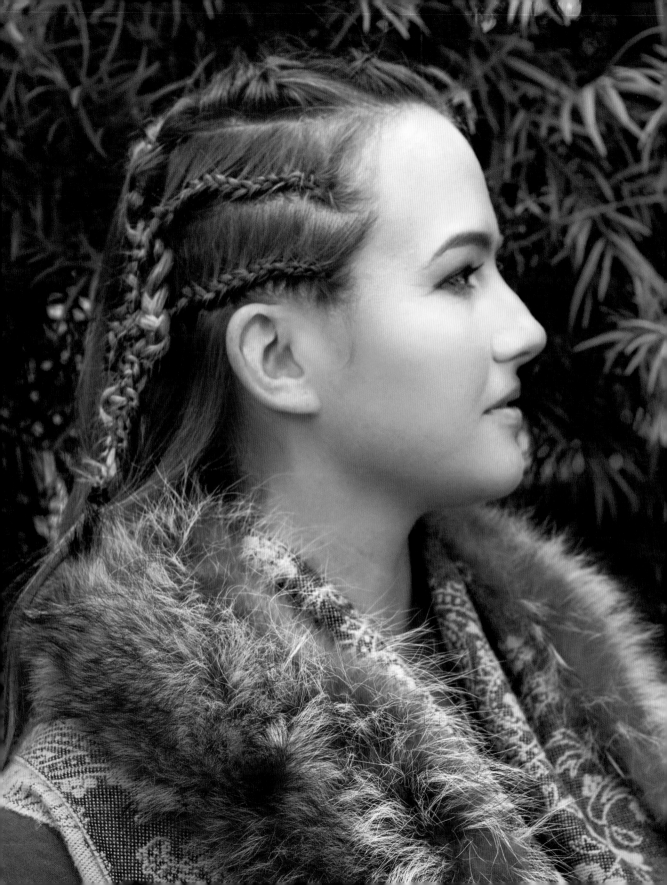

CHAPTER 2

VIKING WARRIORS

In Norse mythology, beautiful hair is a symbol of fertility. Sif, the goddess of fertility and family, had long golden hair representing bountiful wheat. In one story recorded by the Icelandic historian Snorri Sturluson in his *Prose Edda* (ca. 1220), the mischievous god Loki cuts off Sif's hair and is punished severely: not only does he have to make Sif a golden headdress, but he is also forced to offer gifts to three other gods—one of which is Thor's mighty hammer.

Clearly, hair was an important indicator of social status and marital eligibility among the Vikings, and interest in the culture is experiencing a renaissance of sorts thanks to *Vikings*, the History Channel's hit television series. In this chapter I will be demonstrating how to recreate the hairstyles of some leading characters in *Vikings*, including chieftain **Ragnar Lothbrok**—who is based on the legendary Norse hero from the Völsunga saga—as well as **Kwenthrith, Queen of Mercis,** and the Viking shieldmaidens **Lagertha** and **Torvi.** Also included is a hairstyle of the Saxon warrior **Uhtred of Bebbanburg,** the fictional protagonist of the BBC's historical drama series *The Last Kingdom*, which is set during the Viking occupation of England in the ninth century.

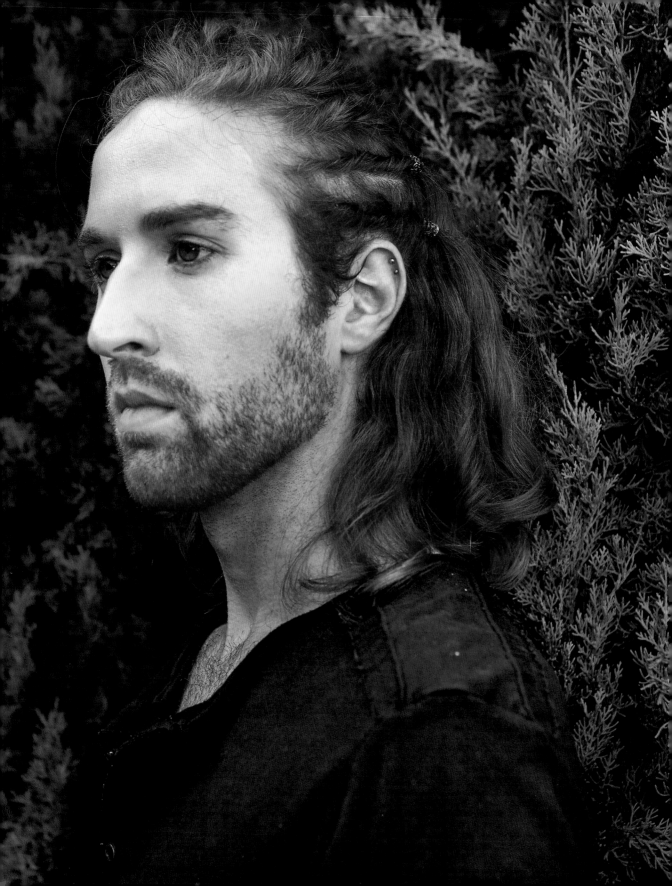

Uhtred OF BEBBANBURG

Most of the action in *The Last Kingdom*—which is based on Bernard Cornwell's bestselling *Saxon Stories* novels—is set during the violent second half of the ninth century, as King Alfred the Great (849–899) unites the separate kingdoms of England against the Viking invaders. Played by German-born actor Alexander Dreymon, Uhtred is captured as a youth at York in 866 by the Danes and raised by their warlord, Ragnar the Fearless. He develops a great love for his Viking comrades, as well as their gods and customs, so when he flees to Wessex following his adoptive family's murder and joins the Saxon army, he has to contend with conflicting loyalties to both the Saxons and the Danes.

SKILL LEVEL: Easy
TIME: 10 minutes

MATERIALS NEEDED:

Hairspray or texture spray

Hair clips

1 small hair elastic

4 small, clear hair elastics

4 silver hair beads

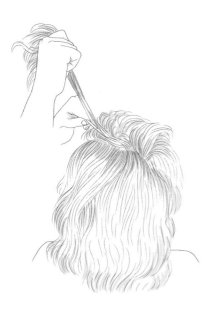

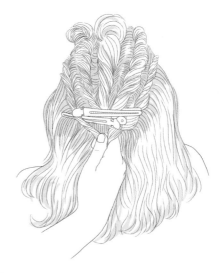

1. To prep the hair for the rough warrior look, tease the hair on top of the head.

2. Now divide the hair on top of the head into five sections, running from the forehead back to the crown. The outermost sections should start at the corners of the forehead, with the other three in between. Liberally spray this hair with hairspray or texture spray so that it will hold its shape better. Twist each of these sections, starting with just a little bit of hair at the forehead. Add in more hair to each twist as you progress back to the crown. Clip the twists for now.

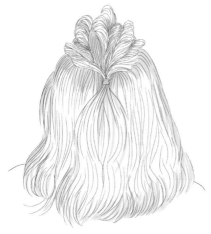

3. Bring the two outermost twists together at the back of the head and secure with a small hair elastic. Let the three other twists hang loose under this.

BEHIND THE SCENES

The character of Uhtred is based partly on Uhtred the Bold, the historical earl of the Kingdom of Northumbria from 1006 to 1016, who led an army into battle at Durham in northeast England and came away with a decisive victory over Malcolm II of Scotland.

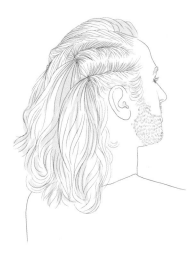

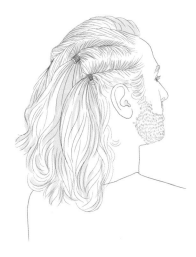

4. Divide the hair on one side of the head in half horizontally, and then make two more twists with each of these halves, securing each twist with a small, clear hair elastic near the back of the head. Repeat this step on the other side of the head.

5. Slide a hair bead over each elastic on the four side twists.

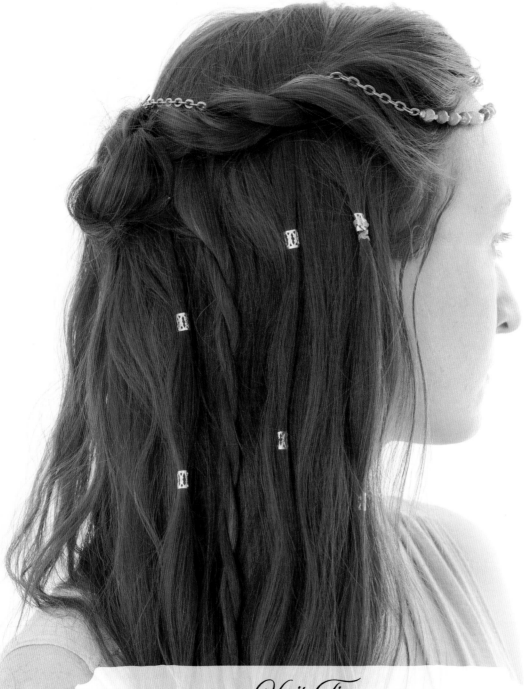

Hair Tip

If your hair is very long, don't worry about making a bun out of the entire length
of the braids—you can let the ends hang free and just remove the elastics.

Kwenthrith

QUEEN OF MERCIA

Kwenthrith enters the action of *Vikings* in season two. Her character is inspired by the powerful, jealous sister of Saint Kenelm and daughter of Kenwulf, King of Mercia (present-day English Midlands) from the ninth-century. Played by American actress Amy Bailey, Kwenthrith seduces Ragnar (page 45), King Ecbert of Wessex, and his son, Aethelwulf, in her quest for supreme power. In addition to her sex appeal, Kwenthrith relies on her natural ruthlessness and superior cunning to dispose of adversaries and protect her throne.

This alluring look comes from episode nine of season two, when a number of Vikings decide to volunteer as mercenaries in Kwenthrith's army.

SKILL LEVEL: Easy
TIME: 15 minutes

MATERIALS NEEDED:
2 small hair elastics
18 silver hair beads
Bobby pins
Necklace or circlet

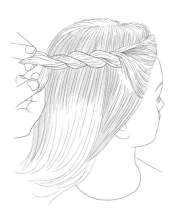

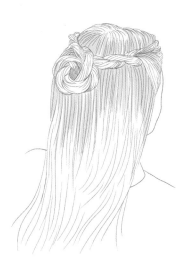

1. Part the hair in the center and grab a large section of hair on either side of the part. Rope-braid each of these sections toward the back of the head and tie them off with an elastic for now.

2. Form these rope braids into a little bun at the back of the head. Pin in place with bobby pins.

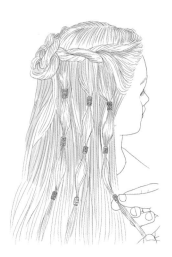

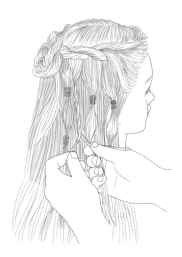

3. Pick up three small sections of hair on each side of the head. Slide three small hair beads onto each one of these sections.

4. Make a small rope accent braid on each side of the head as well, securing them with hair elastics or letting them hang free if you wish to have a looser look. For the finishing touch, drape a beaded necklace or circlet across the forehead and pin it into the rope braids to hold it in place.

Ragnar LOTHBROK

The Norse king Ragnar Lothbrok is more a figure out of folklore than history; there's a saga in which he marries and has four sons (Ubbe, Hvitserk, Sigurd Snake-Eye, and Ivar the Boneless) with Auslag, daughter of the legendary dragonslayer Sigurd and Valkyrie shieldmaiden Brynhildr. The *Vikings* character Ragnar, played by Australian actor Travis Fimmel, has a son with his first wife, Lagertha (page 53), before coming under the spell of the beautiful Auslag. As Earl of Kattegat in southern Norway, he leads his clan on terrifying raids in England and France while struggling to keep them united with one another.

The hairstyle shown here is his classic look from season one.

SKILL LEVEL: Intermediate
TIME: 20 minutes

MATERIALS NEEDED:

3 small hair elastics
Several large hair elastics

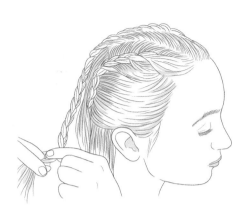

1. Section off the top portion of the hair by making a part, starting at each corner of the forehead and running back to the crown. Divide this section of hair into three subsections. French-braid each of these subsections, finishing the braids to the ends and securing them with small hair elastics.

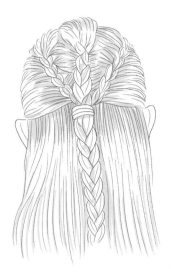

2. Gather up these braids, along with some free-hanging hair at the sides of the head, and tie them into a half ponytail at the back of the head with a large hair elastic.

{ BEHIND THE SCENES

While there are few historical references to how the Vikings styled their hair, the hairstylists on the History Channel show like to imagine what could be done using only period-appropriate hairstyling tools. Thus, you won't find any hair elastics or bobby pins on the actors! Instead, braids are secured either with string or by back-combing the ends so that they stay in place. To create complex updos, gilded thread and a blunt needle are used to sew braids to the head. And if you want to accessorize like these Vikings, you should take a trip to Italy—interviews with cast and crew reveal that many of the hair decorations seen on the show are antique necklaces and jewelry from Italian opera houses!

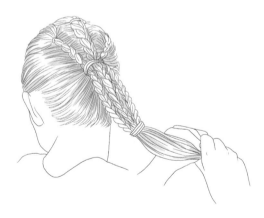

3. Gather this ponytail, along with the remaining hair, into a low ponytail, tying it all together with a large hair elastic (or leather cord, if you want to be authentic!). Then add more hair elastics, spaced a few inches apart, down the length of the ponytail.

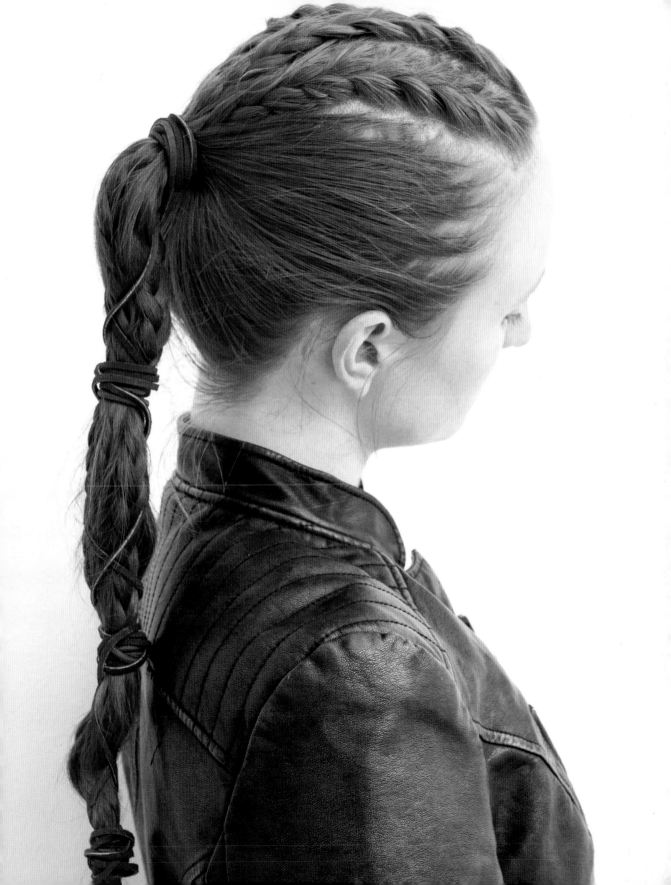

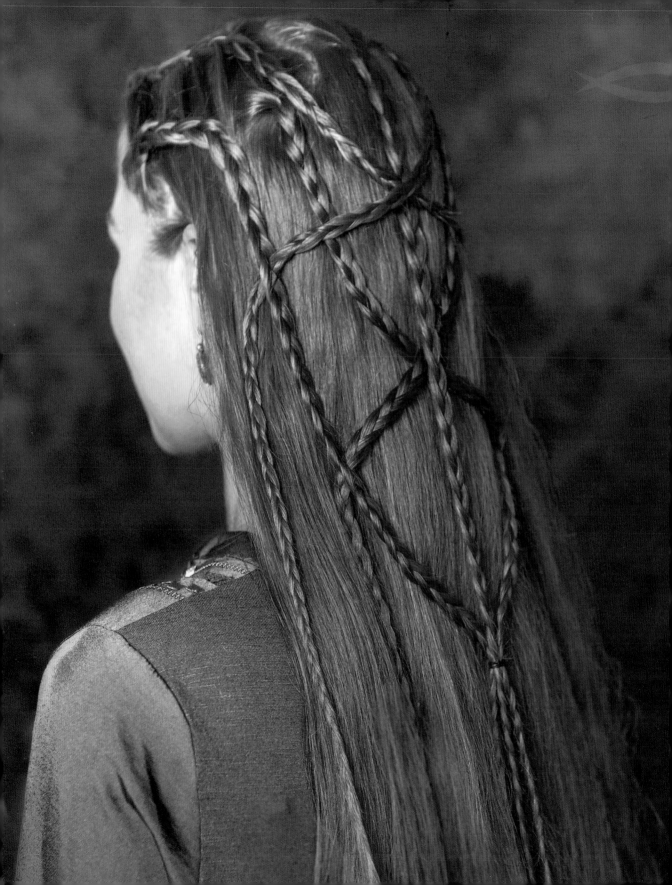

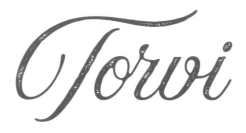

Played by the English actress Georgia Hirst, Torvi is a strong-willed woman. After her first husband, Earl Borg, is brutally executed by Ragnar Lothbrok (page 45), she is forced to murder her abusive second husband, Erlendur, in order to save the life of her lover (and Ragnar's son), Bjorn. Before long she is married to Bjorn and leading battles as a shieldmaiden, second in command under Bjorn's mother, Lagertha (page 53).

Torvi also has some of the most eye-catching and unique hairstyles in the show. The look shown here is from the fourth episode of season four, when Bjorn asks Torvi to be with him instead of Erlendur.

SKILL LEVEL: Intermediate
TIME: 20 minutes

MATERIALS NEEDED:
7 small, clear hair elastics (optional)
1 small hair elastic

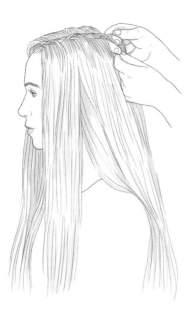

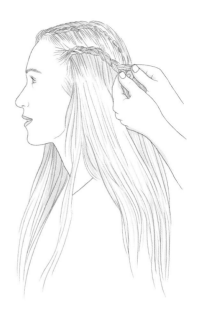

I. Make a center part, and then create a Dutch lace waterfall braid with a 1-inch-wide (2.5 cm) section of hair on each side of the part (see page 17 for instructions on waterfall braiding). Add in hair to the top strands of the braid as you form it toward the back of the head, and remove hair from the bottom strands so that this hair waterfalls out below the braid. When you get to the back of the head, stop adding in new hair and English-braid them to the ends, tying them off with small elastics. (Technically, Torvi doesn't wear hair elastics because these long braids can hold themselves, but you can secure the ends if you want.)

2. Make two more Dutch lace braids below the first ones, one on either side of the head, adding in the hair that came out of the first two waterfall braids. As with the previous braids, stop adding in more hair when you reach the back of the head and English-braid them to the ends, securing these braids with hair elastics.

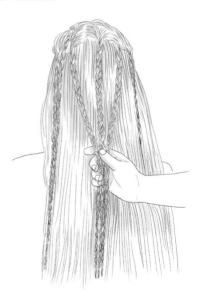

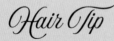

Hair Tip

The *Vikings* show stylists like to "free-style" the characters' looks a lot—they'll have a general concept but make improvisations on it from scene to scene, like a jazz solo. Feel free to make adjustments to fit your whims, too!

3. Now make three small English braids at the back of the head: one at the end of the center part and the other two each starting between the two pairs of Dutch lace braids. Finish these braids to the ends and tie them off.

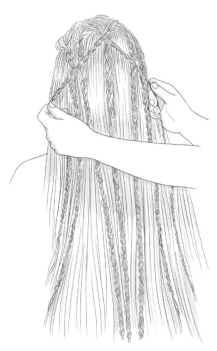

4. Take the tails of the two Dutch lace waterfall braids and cross them at the back of the head, over the center English braid. Then thread these braids through the strands of the two Dutch lace braids. Use a topsy tail to do this or poke your fingers through the Dutch lace braids to pull the others through.

5. Now, cross the two outer English braids under the center English braid. As with the Dutch lace waterfall braids, thread these braids through the two Dutch lace braids.

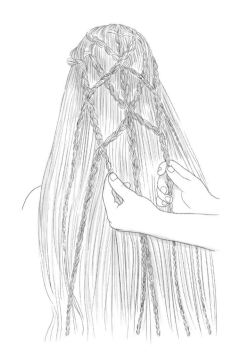

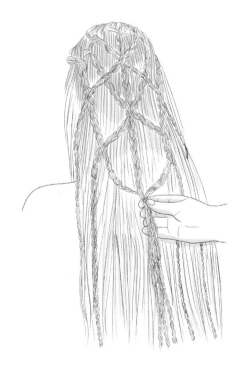

6. Gather up the ends of the center English braid and the Dutch lace braids and tie them together with a small hair elastic.

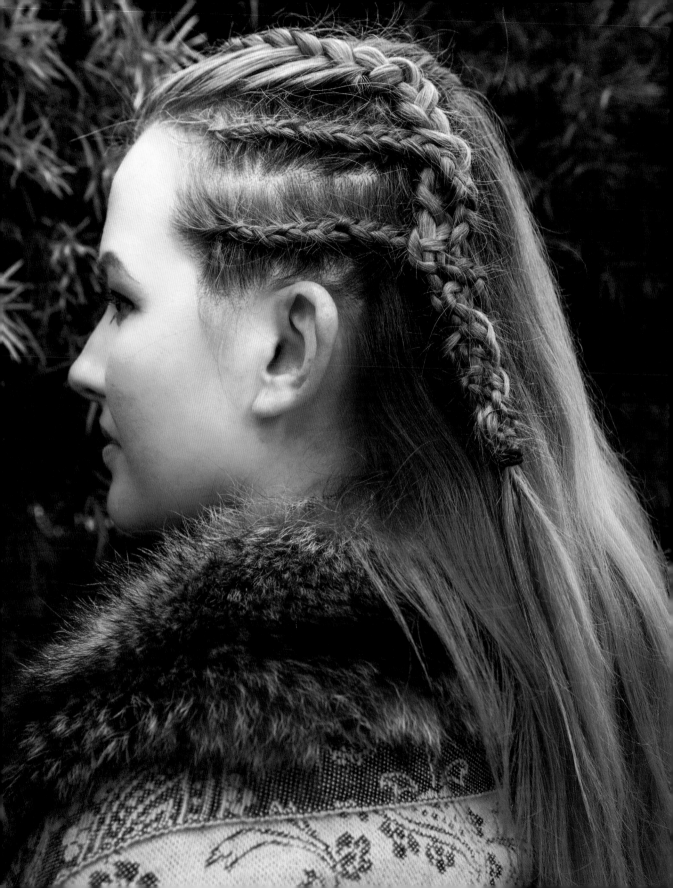

Inspired by

VIKINGS

Lagertha

Played by the Canadian actress Katheryn Winnick, the character of Lagertha is a shieldmaiden and the first wife of Ragnar Lothbrok (page 45). The Lagertha of folklore is believed to have lived in the ninth century, and she appears in the twelfth-century writings of Saxo Grammaticus as "Ladgerda, a skilled Amazon, who, though a maiden, had the courage of a man, and fought in front among the bravest with her hair loose over her shoulders. All marveled at her matchless deeds, for her lock flying down her back betrayed that she was a woman."

The *Vikings* stylists gave Lagertha many awesome looks to live up to this description. The one shown here can be seen in season two, when she has become an earl following her separation from Ragnar.

SKILL LEVEL: Intermediate
TIME: 20 minutes

MATERIALS NEEDED:
8 small hair elastics
Hair clips

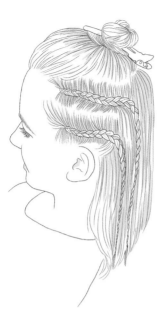

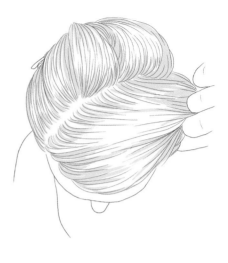

I. ◆ Gather all the hair on top of the head and clip it out of the way for now. On one side of the head, divide the hair into two horizontal halves. Create Dutch lace braids with these two sections, starting at the front of the head and going backward. When you reach the back of the head, English-braid them to the ends and secure with small hair elastics. Repeat this step on the other side of the head.

2. ◆ Let down the top section of hair and draw a slightly diagonal part, extending from near the front of the head on one side to near the back of the head on the other side.

{ BEHIND THE SCENES

The hairstyles in *Vikings* act as a device for character development. For instance, the progression of Ragnar's hairstyles mimics the progression of his character: the more power and weight of responsibility he accumulated, the more hair weight he chopped off, until at his zenith he had no hair at all. Lagertha rose in power as well, but her hair became ever more complicated in the process. These structured styles serve a shieldmaiden's purpose, keeping hair out of the eyes and intimidating the enemy, so when she became an earl, perhaps she was intentionally using her hairstyles to amplify her martial might and make sure everyone remembers how she took her power in the first place.

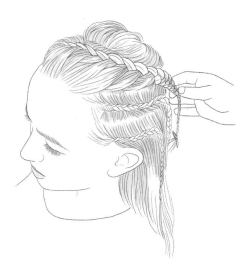

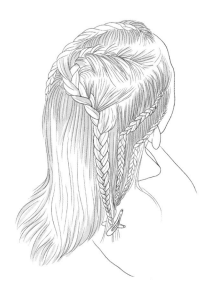

3. French-braid the hair in front of the part, starting at the front and going backward in a diagonal so that the end of the braid falls behind one ear. Secure with an elastic to hold the braid in place.

4. Now French-braid the hair behind the part at an opposite diagonal, finishing off the braid behind the opposite ear.

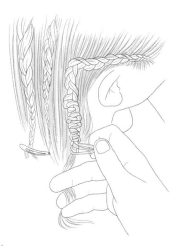

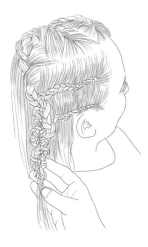

5. Turn all six braids into "slide-up" braids—that is, remove the elastic at the ends, grab the end of one strand, and slide the other two strands up toward the head until they can go no farther.

6. Loosen the slide-up braids a little bit and then secure them with the small hair elastics. Then gently braid together the three braids on each side of the head, securing each larger braid with an elastic.

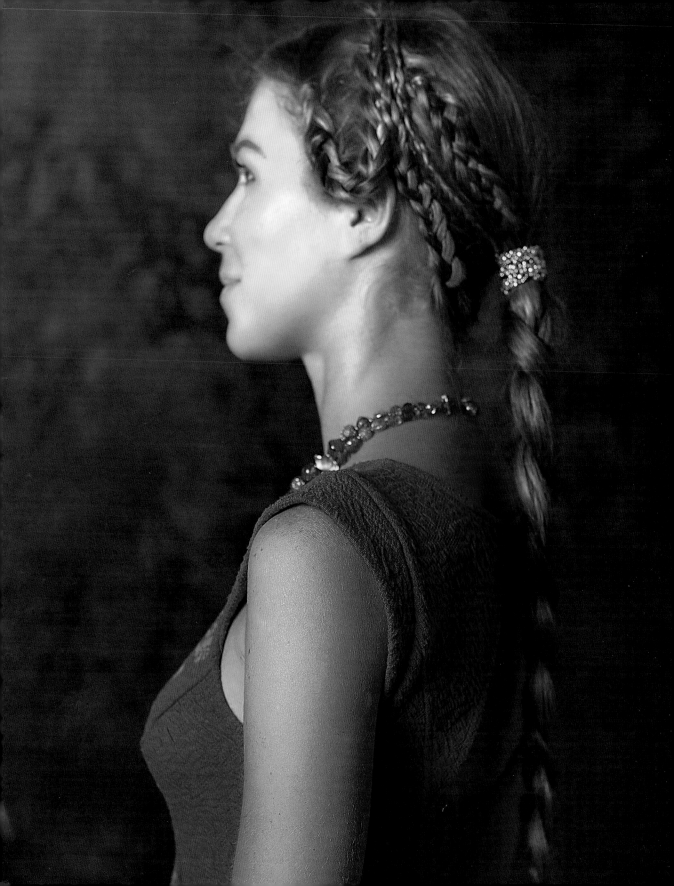

CHAPTER 3

Renaissance Royals

As in other eras of history, the way Renaissance women wore their hair was strongly connected to social status and religious observance. In this chapter we will be recreating hairstyles from four historical dramas set in Renaissance Britain, France, and Italy. As this cultural apex is flourishing in fifteenth-century Florence, we are introduced to the inner rivalries of a notorious aristocratic family, including those of the clever and beautiful **Lucrezia Borgia**, in the Showtime drama series *The Borgias*. The 2017 Starz miniseries *The White Princess* transports us to England in 1486, where two warring houses are united by the marriage of King Henry VII and **Elizabeth of York**. Showtime's *The Tudors* examines the scandalous life of Henry VII and Elizabeth's son, King Henry VIII, who beheaded two of his six wives—including the vivacious, tempestuous **Anne Boleyn**—and initiated the English Reformation in the process. The TV series *Reign*, which first aired in 2013, follows **Mary, Queen of Scots's** ascent to power in Scotland and France in the late sixteenth century, as well as her growing rivalry with Queen Elizabeth I of England.

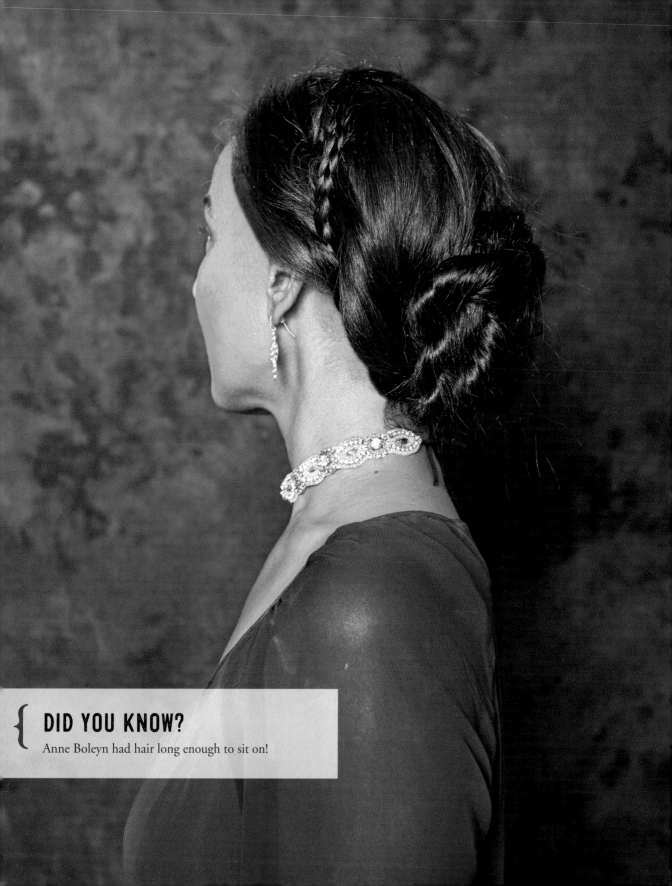

Anne BOLEYN

In 1536, after being accused of adultery with multiple men, Anne Boleyn became the first English queen to be publicly executed. Reportedly fond of wine, archery, and gambling, young Anne was described by witnesses as sharp-tongued and flirtatious. In 1526, while serving as a lady-in-waiting to Queen Catherine, Henry VIII's first wife, she caught the eye of the king, eventually giving birth to Queen Elizabeth I and setting into motion one of the most dramatic series of events in English history.

In the Showtime historical drama *The Tudors*, she is skillfully portrayed by the English actress Natalie Dormer. This updo can be seen on Anne at the end of season two, as she fights to hold on to her crown.

SKILL LEVEL: Easy
TIME: 10 minutes

MATERIALS NEEDED:

3 small hair elastics
Bobby pins

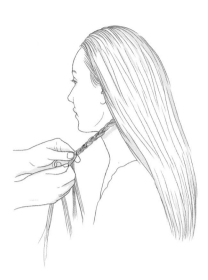

1. Make a center part, and then gather two small sections of hair from the nape of the neck. English-braid these sections and secure at the ends.

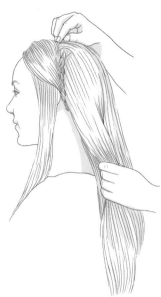

2. Wrap each of these braids around each side of the head and across the top, pinning them in place. Make sure to leave out strips of hair (about 2 inches, or 5 cm, wide) that frame the face on both sides.

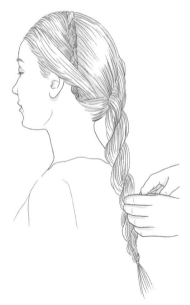

3. Gather the remaining hair, including the hair framing the face, at the base of the head and rope-braid it. Secure the ends with a hair elastic.

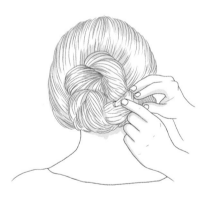

4. Form this braid into a circle at the back of the head and pin it in place with bobby pins.

REIGN

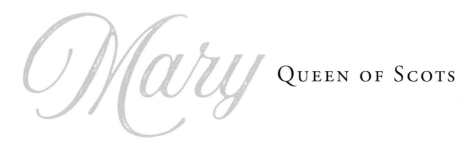 Queen of Scots

Becoming queen when she was only six days old, Mary, Queen of Scots lived a short life full of political intrigue, scandal, and murder before she was beheaded in 1587 at the command of her rival to the English throne, Queen Elizabeth I. *Reign* (somewhat inaccurately) follows the early period of Mary's life at the French court of Henry II, during her marriage to King Francis, and later in Scotland as she attempted to secure her own crown.

This particular hairstyle is from season one, during Mary's days at the French court.

SKILL LEVEL: Easy
TIME: 15 minutes

MATERIALS NEEDED:

3 small hair elastics
Bobby pins
Tiara (optional)

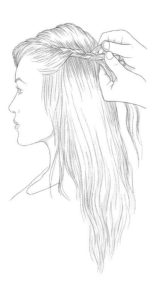

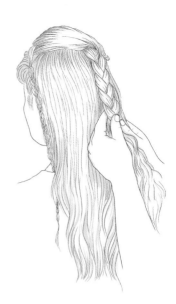

1. Make a center part, then gather a small section of hair at the front of the head on one side of the part. Lace-braid this section, adding in just three small sections of new hair from the front hairline at the top of the forehead. English-braid it to the ends and secure with a small hair elastic. Repeat this step on the other side of the head.

2. Gather up the hair at the crown of the head and English-braid it, securing the ends with a small hair elastic.

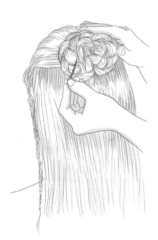

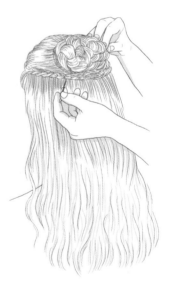

3. Coil the English braid around itself at the crown to make a bun. Pin to hold the braid in place.

4. Wrap each small lace braid around the bun (wrapping along the bottom of the bun, then over), and tuck the ends of the braids underneath the bun, pinning to secure them. If you have a tiara, place it directly in front of the bun.

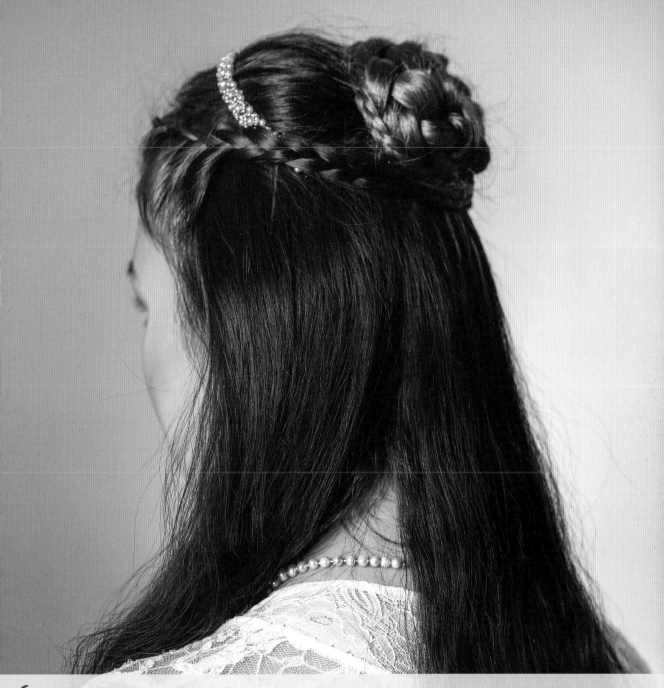

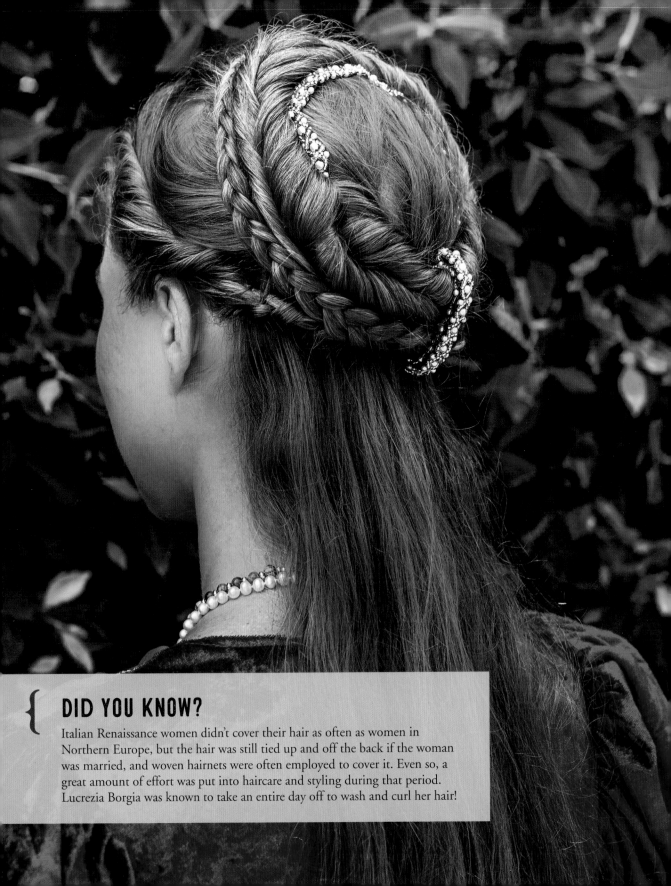

Inspired by

THE BORGIAS

Lucrezia BORGIA

Born into the infamous Borgia family, Lucrezia (1480–1519) was most likely used as a pawn in her family's quest to take over parts of Italy. Her father, Pope Alexander VI, arranged for all three of her politically advantageous marriages, the first one occurring when Lucrezia was only thirteen. He also helped end her marriages when they were no longer beneficial to the family. Yet this cunning, golden-haired femme fatale—played by the English actress Holliday Grainger in the shocking historical drama *The Borgias*—had a power all her own.

The hairstyle shown here can be seen in a scene from season two, when Lucrezia is meeting with her lover Paolo.

SKILL LEVEL: Intermediate
TIME: 20 minutes

MATERIALS NEEDED:

Bobby pins
4 small hair elastics
Hair clips
Curling iron (optional)
Decorative ribbon
Tiara

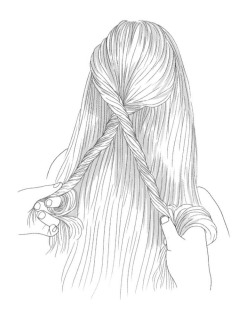

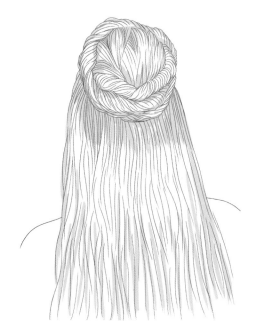

1. Make a center part, and then take two sections of hair at the back of the head and twist them.

2. Form these twists into a circle at the upper back of the head and pin them in place.

Hair Tip

Curly and wavy hair work best for this style! The texture helps hold the twists together and keeps the bobby pins from sliding out. So, if you are not blessed with natural waves or curls, take a curling iron and add some curls to your hair before you begin.

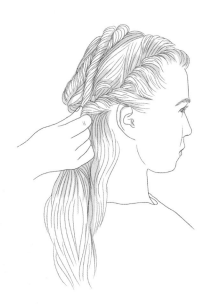

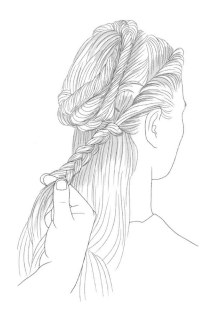

3. On one side of the head, gather a 2-inch-wide (5 cm) section of hair around the face, and twist it until you reach about ear level, clipping it in place. Repeat this step on the other side of the head.

4. English-braid the hair below the clip on both sides and secure with small hair elastics.

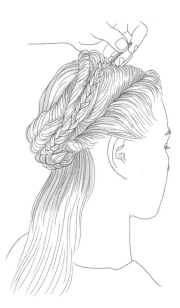

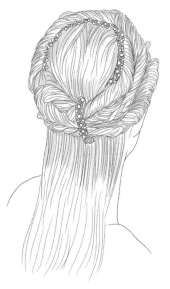

5. Wrap these braids around the outside of the circle you made earlier, pinning them in place.

6. Take the decorative ribbon and pin it over the bottom of the circle. Then position more decorative ribbon or a tiara inside the top of the circle.

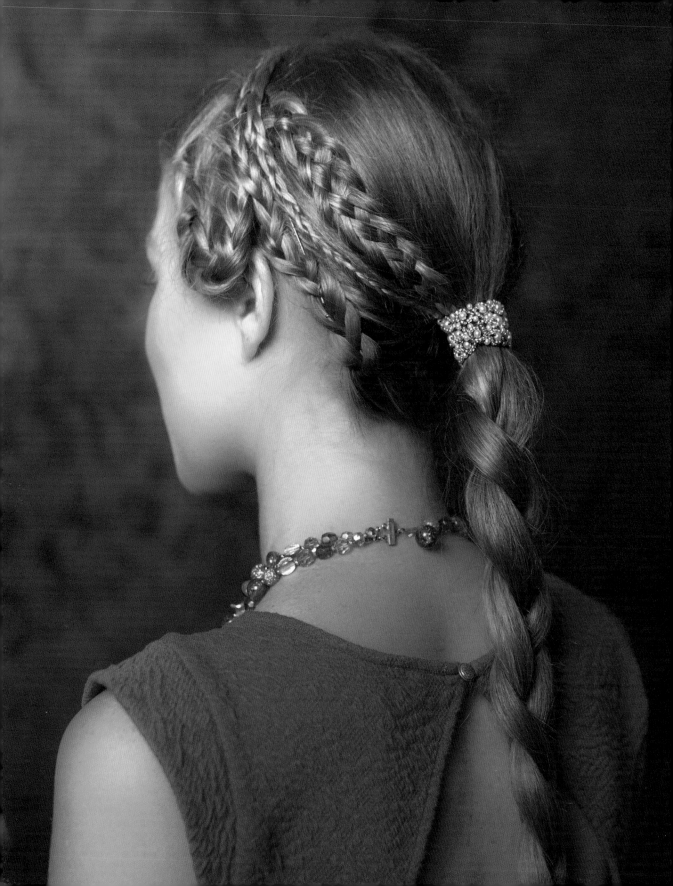

THE WHITE PRINCESS

Elizabeth OF YORK

When Elizabeth of York married Henry VII in 1486, their union represented the end of the Wars of the Roses. A mother of seven children, of whom only four survived past childhood—including the extravagant and vengeful Tudor monarch Henry VIII (see page 59)—the historical Elizabeth of York wasn't exactly badass in the traditional sense. In fact, she was known as a gentle, doting wife and mother, avoiding politics and enjoying the company of her pet greyhounds until her untimely death on her 37th birthday in 1503. Based on the historical fiction novel by Philippa Gregory, the Showtime miniseries *The White Princess* cast English actress Jodie Comer in the lead role and presented a much saucier version of known events.

SKILL LEVEL: Advanced
TIME: 20 minutes

MATERIALS NEEDED:

Hair clips

2 small hair elastics

Hair extensions (optional)

2 large hair elastics

Decorative ribbon

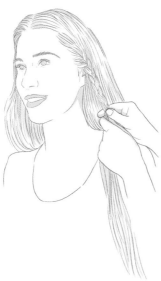

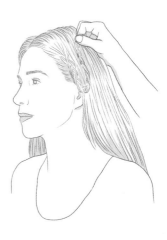

I. Make a center part, and then gather a section of hair on one side of the head, in front of the ears. At about eyebrow level, start lace-braiding this hair. Lace-braid in the rest of the hair along the side hairline until you get to the ear, and then English-braid it to the ends and secure with a small hair elastic. Repeat this step on the other side of the head.

2. Fold one of these braids in half so that the braid length is now pointing up to the top of the head.

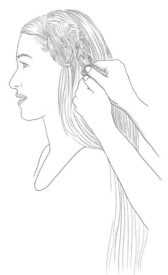

3. At the same height where you started the braid, weave in a fourth and fifth strand of hair like you would in a five-strand braid pattern (page 19). Repeat this step with the braid on the other side of the head. Finish these braids to the ends and clip them in place.

Hair Tip

Many historical and fantasy women's styles use small braids around the face. For people with bangs, this can be an issue. To work with bangs, use styles with French or lace braids so you can start the braid near the face, but add in longer hair from farther back so that the braid can continue. If the style has a headband-like braid or a high bun, you can also brush the bangs back and pin them underneath these parts of the style.

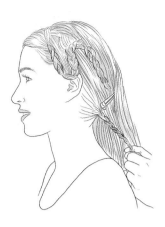

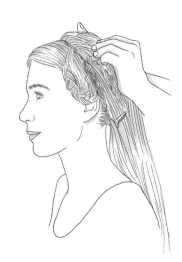

4. If the hair is long and somewhat thick, gather some hair from the nape of the neck and English-braid it to the ends. If the hair is shorter, make two English braids—one on each side of the neck—or make a longer braid out of a length of hair extensions.

5. Wrap the rope braids or hair extension braid around the side and over the top of the head, pinning it in place. It should lie on top of the five-strand braids, holding them tight against the head.

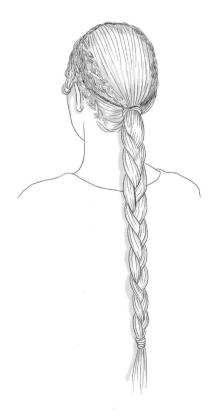

6. Now gather all the hair, including the five-strand braids, and tie it into a low ponytail, securing it with the large hair elastic. Undo any braiding below this hair elastic, and then English-braid the entire ponytail, securing it with another hair elastic. Finally, wrap the decorative ribbon around the top ponytail elastic.

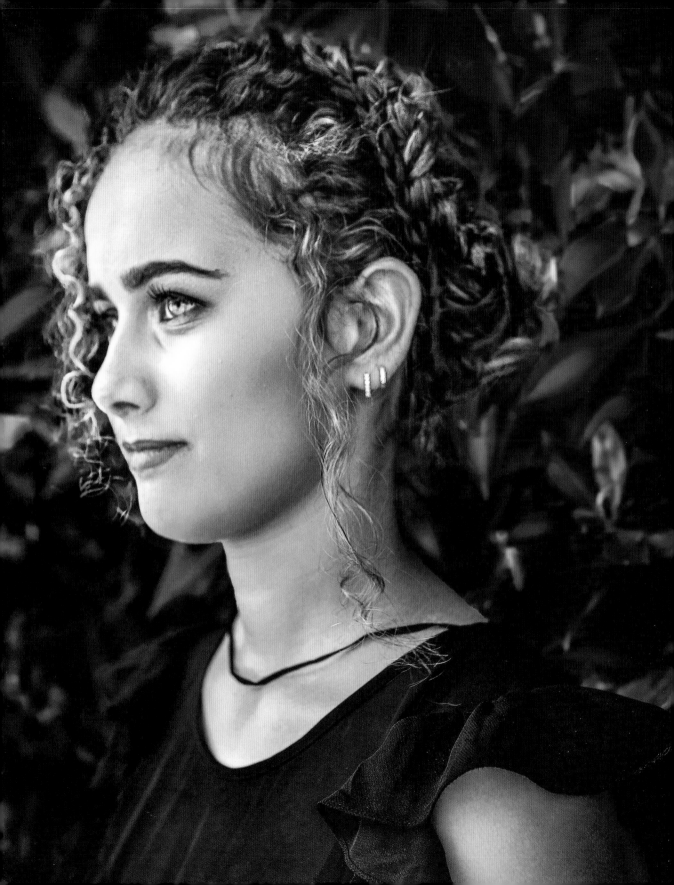

CHAPTER 4

ROMANTIC RENEGADES

In this chapter, I have recreated hairstyles from movies and TV shows that depict the romance and adventure of the eighteenth and nineteenth centuries, including *Black Sails*, *Penny Dreadful*, *Outlander*, and the 2005 movie *Pride and Prejudice*. *Black Sails* is a pirate adventure drama set in the early eighteenth century (ca. 1715) in the lawless West Indies, where ruthless and greedy buccaneers are engaged in a bloody contest over the region's wealth. One of these pirates is **Charles Vane**, a former slave and protégé of Blackbeard who establishes himself as one of the most feared captains in the Caribbean. Vane's temporary captive, **Max**, is another former slave who—like Vane—vies for the love of the powerful black marketeer Eleanor Guthrie. Set in Victorian London (ca. 1891), *Penny Dreadful* centers on the gifted but tortured figure of **Vanessa Ives**, who uses her mystic powers to vanquish evil spirits. The time-travelling drama *Outlander*, based on the bestselling historical-fantasy book series by Diana Gabaldon, follows the unlikely romance between a twentieth-century combat nurse and an eighteenth-century Scottish fugitive, both of whom owe their lives in part to the latter's older sister, **Jenny Murray**. Based on the beloved early nineteenth-century novel by Jane Austen, the 2005 film adaptation of *Pride and Prejudice* follows the story of **Lizzy Bennet**, a sharp-witted rebel against the rigid expectations of Regency-era British society.

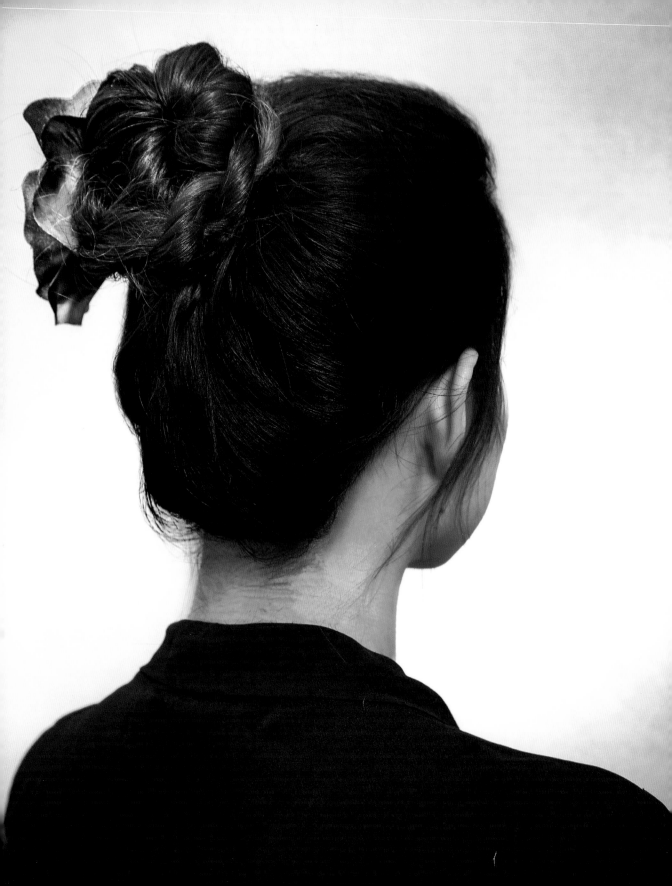

Vanessa Ives

Brilliantly played by the French actress Eva Green, the medium Vanessa Ives is a standout original among a cast of characters culled from Gothic literature, including *Frankenstein*, *Dracula*, *The Picture of Dorian Gray*, and *The Strange Case of Dr. Jekyll and Mr. Hyde*. Ives's mysterious background and literal inner demons play center stage in this horror drama, which is inspired by the cheap, sensational stories common in Victorian London—"penny dreadful" was a nickname for serial stories on fantastical topics that you could buy for a penny.

This fashionable style is a variation on the Newport Knot, a twisted updo that was popular in England around the turn of the twentieth century. (That's a little later than the Victorian era, but close enough!)

SKILL LEVEL: Easy
TIME: 10 minutes

MATERIALS NEEDED:
Teasing comb
Bobby pins
Fabric flower hair accessory

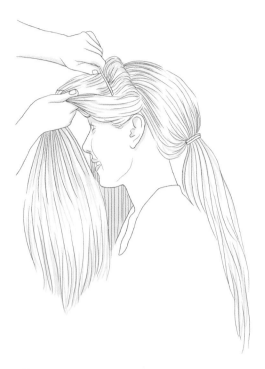

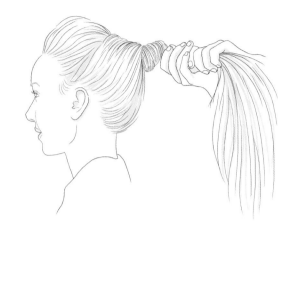

1. Section off the hair along the forehead and side hairlines. Tease this hair to give it volume.

2. Now gently brush all of this hair back and gather it into a high ponytail, tightly twisting up the hair.

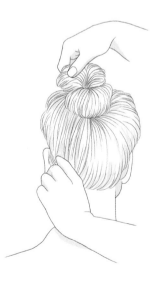

3. Make a loop with the twist so that the loop points upward and the tail passes between the loop and the head. To do this, hold the twist up, then fold it in half so the tail hangs down. Holding the tail steady with one hand, twist the fold once in the direction of the tail. You should now have a loop that you're holding flat against the head. Pin this loop in place.

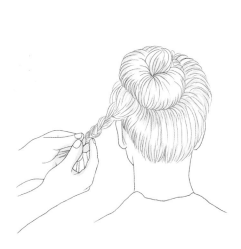

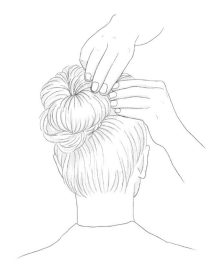

4. Rope-braid the hair tail.

5. Wrap this rope braid around the pinned loop and pin the braid in place. Then place a fabric flower hair accessory on the lower side of the updo.

Hair Tip

If your hair isn't long enough to make both the loop and the rope braid, use all of your hair to make the loop, and then clip some extensions around a large hair elastic. Fit this elastic around the pinned loop made with your own hair and rope-braid the extensions around it.

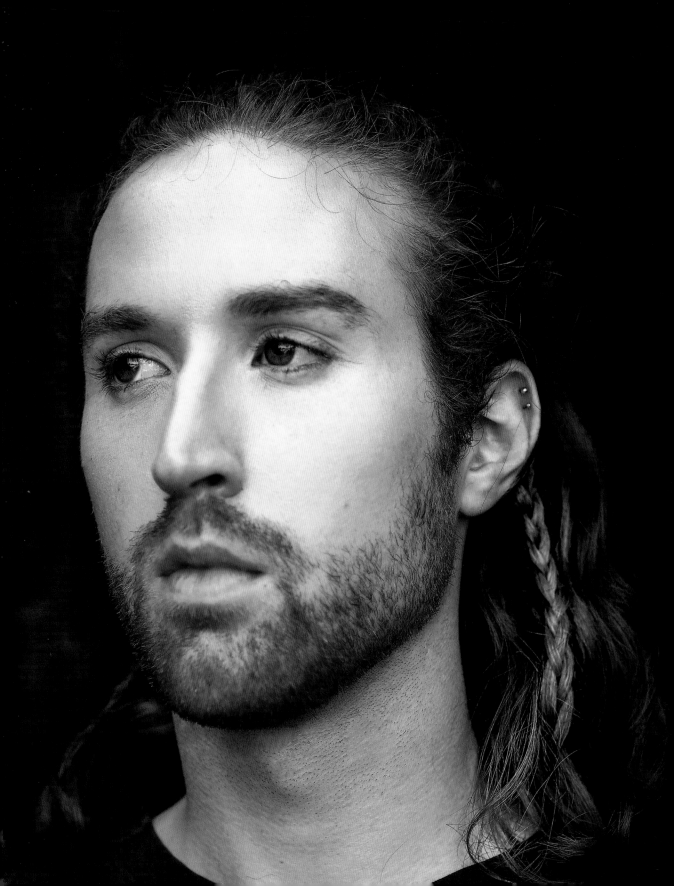

Charles Vane

The character of this fan-favorite swashbuckler is based on the real-life privateer-turned-pirate of the same name, whose heyday of pillaging ranged from 1715 or 1716 to his death by hanging in 1720. Portrayed by the American actor Zach McGowan, Charles Vane is captain of the ship *Ranger* and one of New Providence Island's top pirates.

Charles's style is a simple, no-nonsense look that keeps his long hair out of his face. This is an excellent starter hairstyle for the beginning braider!

SKILL LEVEL: Easy
TIME: 5 minutes

MATERIALS NEEDED:

1 large hair elastic
or suede or leather cord

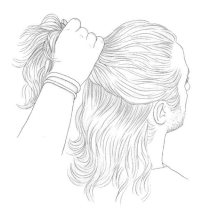

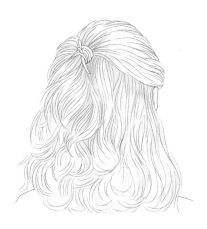

1. Make a horizontal parting through the hair, from ear to ear and across the upper back of the head. Gather up all the hair above this part.

2. Tie this hair into a ponytail with the large hair elastic—use a suede or leather cord to be more authentic.

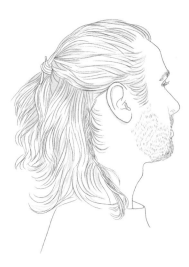

3. Pick up a small section of hair from behind one ear, and English-braid it to the ends. You don't have to secure the ends, because small braids hold themselves together. Repeat this step with a small amount of hair from behind the other ear.

OUTLANDER

Jenny Murray

Outlander is a passionate and nerve-wracking show that blends sci-fi, action, and romance. It takes place in the eighteenth-century Scottish Highlands, where Claire Beauchamp accidentally falls back in time from the twentieth century, falls in love with the fugitive "Red Jamie" Fraser, and then attempts to stop the bloody 1745 Jacobite Rebellion that historically marks the end of the Highland way of life. For this style, we focus on the tough-as-nails Jenny Murray (née Fraser), Jamie's sister, played by the Irish actress Laura Donnelly.

In the books, Jenny (as the "responsible" Fraser sibling) tends toward practical styles and usually wears her hair pinned up under a kerchief like most married women of the time. Luckily for us, though, in the middle of the first season, the show offers a beautiful braided style to recreate!

SKILL LEVEL: Intermediate
TIME: 20 minutes

MATERIALS NEEDED:
3 small hair elastics
Bobby pins

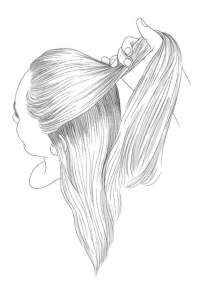

1. Make a part through the hair that runs from ear to ear and up across the crown of the head. Gather the hair on top of this part.

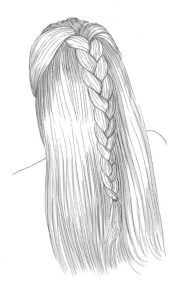

2. English-braid this hair to the ends and secure it with a small hair elastic.

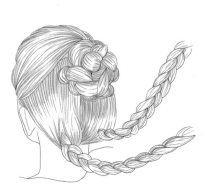

3. Wrap this braid around itself to make a bun at the top of the head. Pin it in place. Divide the remaining hair in half. Braid each half in a three-strand braid, directing the braids upward, so there is no bulging at the roots of the braids when you lift them up to the bun. Secure the braids with small elastics.

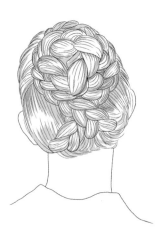

4. Cross these braids at the back of the head and pin them to the opposite sides of the bun. Wrap the remaining tails of the braids around the bun and pin in place. Tuck the tails underneath the lengths of braid that make the X in back so that you don't cover this feature.

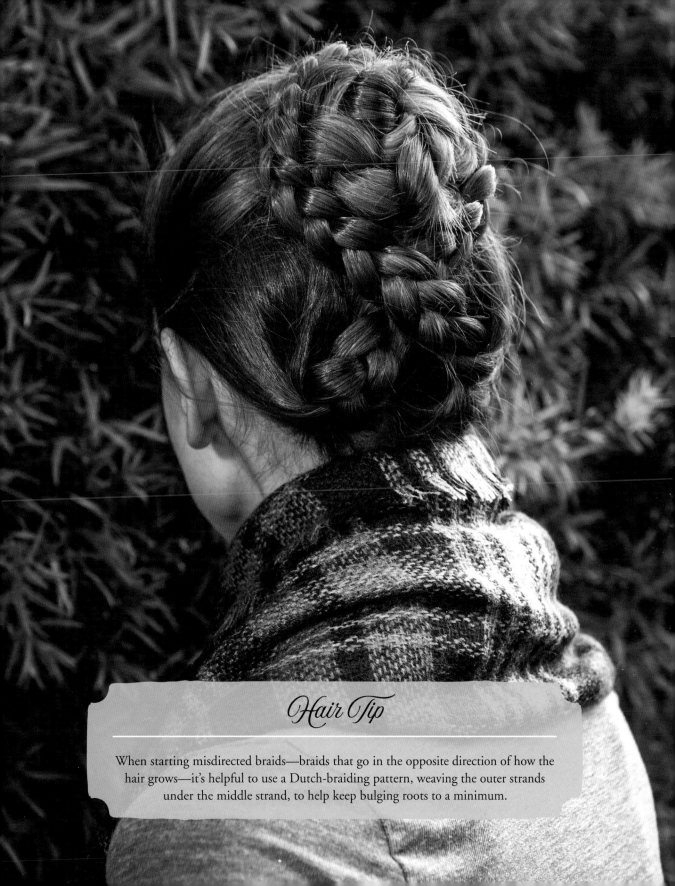

Hair Tip

When starting misdirected braids—braids that go in the opposite direction of how the hair grows—it's helpful to use a Dutch-braiding pattern, weaving the outer strands under the middle strand, to help keep bulging roots to a minimum.

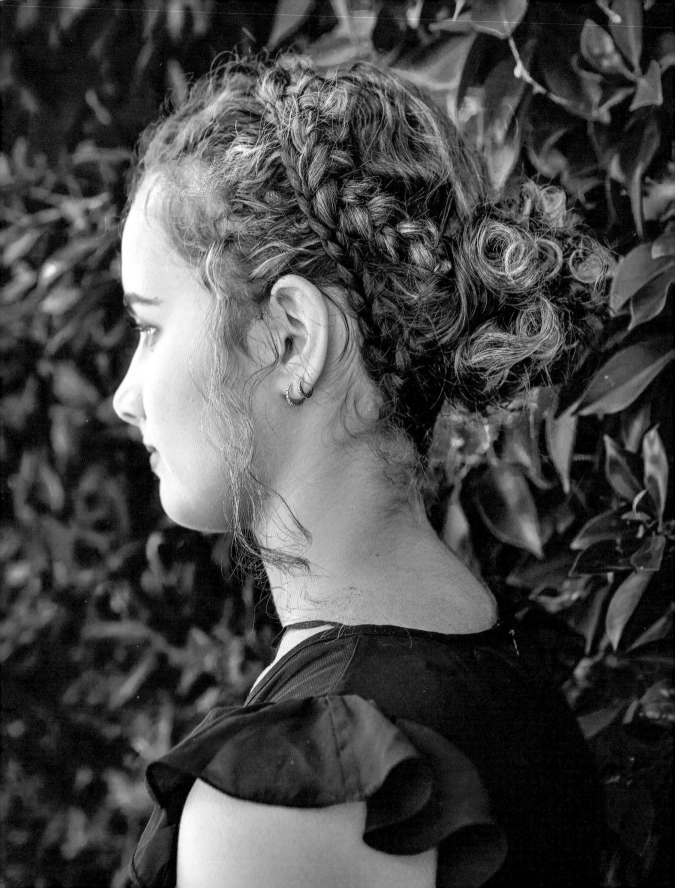

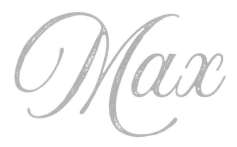

Prostitute-turned-madam Max, played by the Canadian actress Jessica Parker Kennedy, can readily be described as "crafty." Raised in slavery and later captured by the motley crew of Charles Vane (page 79), she is not one to give up as she seeks to become the merchant queen of Nassau.

This style is a version of the look she wears once she's climbed the social ladder and become madam.

SKILL LEVEL: Advanced
TIME: 20 minutes

MATERIALS NEEDED:

Hair clips
3 small hair elastics
Bobby pins
Curling iron (optional)

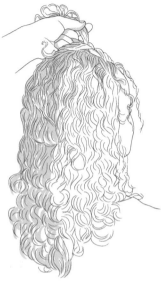

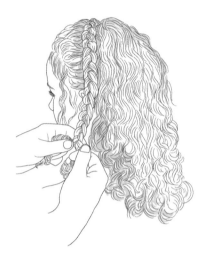

I. Section off some wispy bits of hair around the front hairline and clip them out of the way for now. Starting behind one ear, make a Dutch lace braid pointing upward.

2. Form this braid over the top of the head and around the other side, adding in hair from along the forehead. Stop adding in new hair when you reach the other ear, and finish the braid to the ends. Secure it with a small elastic.

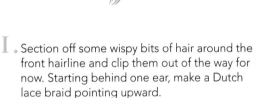

{ DID YOU KNOW?

For much of history, hair has been closely associated with female sexuality. It was considered acceptable for a girl to wear her hair long and loose until she was married, at which point she was expected to start wearing updos in public. Loose hair was reserved for intimate settings. This is why Maxine's hair becomes more elaborate and styled in updos as she transitions from being a prostitute to the more professional brothel madam.

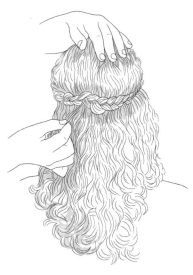

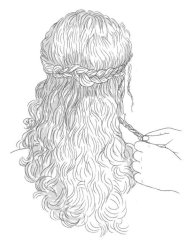

3. Pin the tail of this braid across the back of the head. If it's long enough to reach the beginning of the braid on the other side of the head, pin it parallel to the start of this braid.

4. From one side of the nape of the neck, grab a small section of hair and English-braid it to the ends. Secure it with a small hair elastic. Repeat this step with a small section of hair on the other side of the nape of the neck.

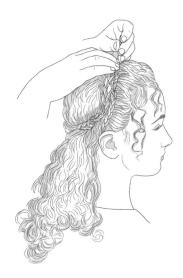

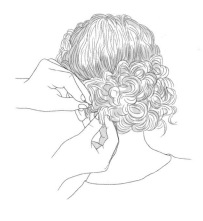

5. Wrap these small braids over the top of the head, in front of the large braid, and pin them in place.

6. If you don't have curly hair, curl the rest of the hair with a curling iron, including the wispy bits at the face. Leaving the wispy bits out, scrunch up the rest of the hair, one large section at a time, and pin into a messy bun at the lower back of the head.

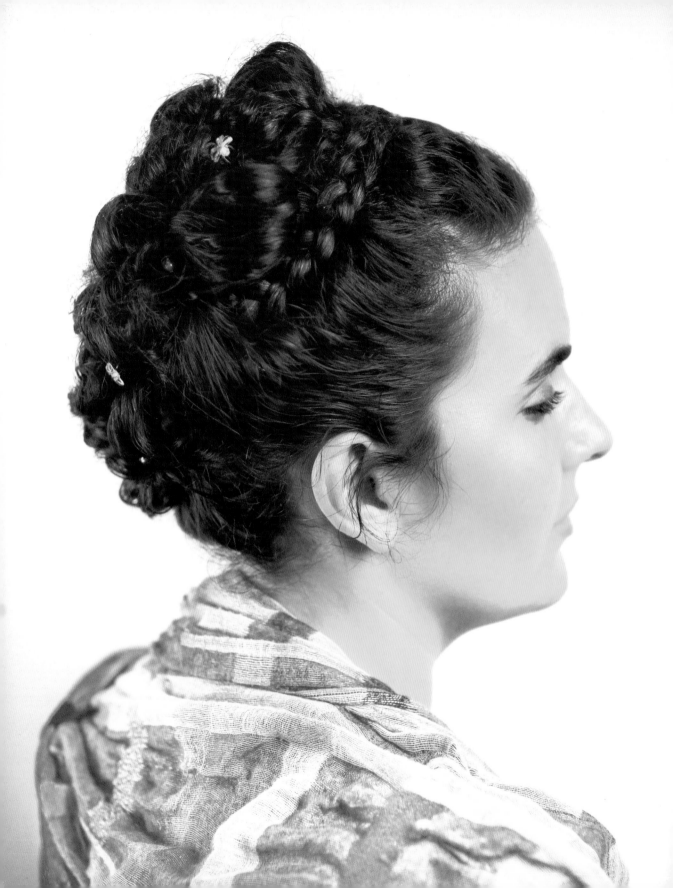

Inspired by

PRIDE AND PREJUDICE

Lizzy Bennet

Played by the English actress Kiera Knightley in the 2005 movie version of *Pride and Prejudice*, Lizzy Bennet is headstrong and independent, and expected to find a wealthy husband. When she matches wits with the arrogant Mr. Darcy, one of the most entertaining and satisfying courtships ever written ensues.

Lizzy wears this fancy pearl-studded style in the ballroom party scene, when she first meets Mr. Darcy.

SKILL LEVEL: Advanced
TIME: 30 minutes

MATERIALS NEEDED:
Hair clips
1 small hair elastic
Bobby pins
Curling iron (optional)
Several pearl hair pins

DID YOU KNOW?

During much of the eighteenth century, large hairstyles were in fashion. Hairdressing shops sold wigs and hairpieces that could easily be pinned to a woman's natural hair with a comb. Women also gathered fallen hair from combs, balled it into clumps, secured those to their heads with hairpins, and then draped their natural hair over the clumps for a more voluminous look. In the Regency era (ca. 1795–1837), hairstyles became less elaborate, but curly hair remained the standard of beauty. Many modest English women wore bonnets when out and about, with ringlets of hair framing the face. At the time, hair was curled with iron rods and clamps heated in the fire—the precursor to our modern hair curlers.

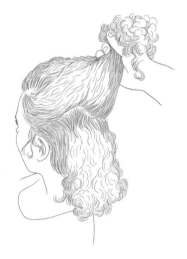

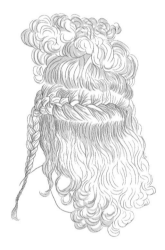

1. Horizontally divide the hair in half.

2. Clip up the top section of the hair for now. Take a horizontal section of hair from the lower half, right below the part, and French-braid this section from one side of the head to the other. When you reach the other side of the head, stop adding in new hair and English-braid it to the ends. Secure the braid with a small hair elastic.

Hair Tip

This braid is meant to wrap around the whole head. If the hair is not long enough to do that, you can make two braids instead, starting in the middle of the back of the head, with each braid ending on opposite sides of the head.

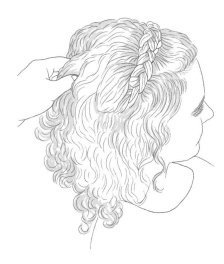

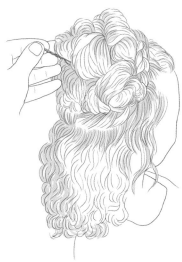

3. Now wrap the braid over the top of the head like a headband and pin it in place.

4. Let down the top half of the hair you clipped up earlier. If you don't have curly hair, curl it with a small curling iron. With small sections at a time, wrap the hair around two fingers to form barrel curls. Pin each of these barrel curls to the head directly behind the headband braid. Make sure to pin the curls close together so that you have a solid mass of curls at the top of the head.

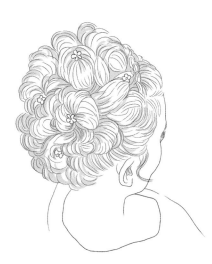

5. Curl the rest of the hair, also making barrel curls like in step 4. Pin these curls along the bottom of the existing curl bun to make it larger and to cover the braid at the back of the head. Finish off the style by inserting pearl hair pins among the curls at various points.

Hair Tip

The actress wore bangs with this style, so if you have bangs, let them hang free!

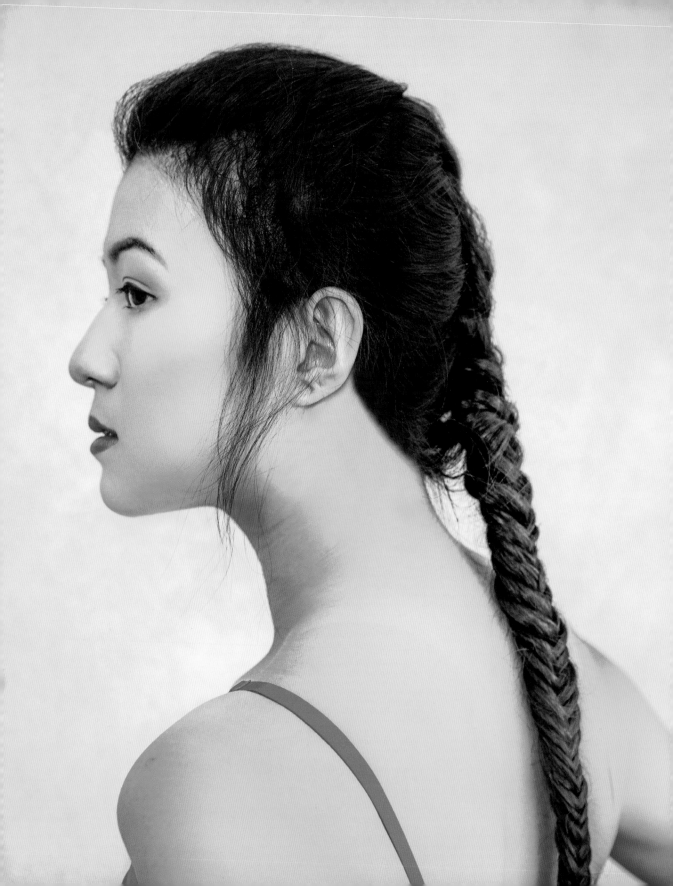

CHAPTER 5

FIERCE FANTASY

Now we leave the world of romance and adventure and enter a realm of fantasy and make-believe. The looks in this chapter—which are inspired by several popular fantasy TV series and films—are more extravagant than the historically inspired styles of the previous chapter, but still heavily inspired by real-world artistic traditions. *Game of Thrones*, which has won multiple Emmys and is based on the book series *A Song of Ice and Fire* (ASOIAF) by George R. R. Martin, has had its fans in a frenzy since its premiere in 2011. This medieval-inspired HBO series follows nine powerful families—whose members include **Cersei Lannister**, **Sansa Stark**, **Margaery Tyrell**, and **Daenerys Targaryen**—as they plot to take over the coveted Iron Throne. Speaking of medieval, BBC's *Merlin* follows the characters of the Arthurian legend as youths, including Arthur's potent nemesis, **Morgana Pendragon**. In *Once Upon a Time*, the residents of Storybrooke, Maine, discover that they are transplants from a fairytale world, and only one woman—the bail-bond agent **Emma Swan**—has the power to break the curse that enslaves them. In *The Shannara Chronicles*, based on the YA book series by Terry Brooks, the world known as the Four Lands is being threatened by demons, and it is up to three young heroes, including the orphan thief **Eretria**, to save it. From the novels of J. R. R. Tolkien come *The Hobbit* and *The Lord of the Rings* film trilogies, where hobbits, wizards, dwarves, and more—including the elves **Legolas** and **Tauriel** and the shieldmaiden **Éowyn**—join forces against the evil creatures and sorcerers within Middle-earth. Finally, **Diana Prince** lends her unparalleled Amazonian fighting prowess to the aid of World War I British troops in the 2017 blockbuster movie *Wonder Woman*.

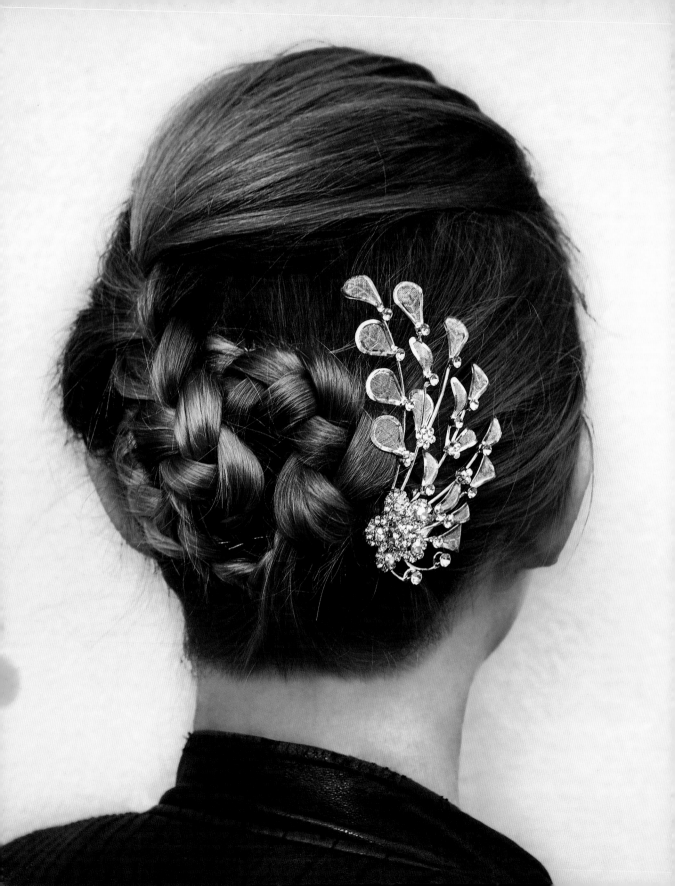

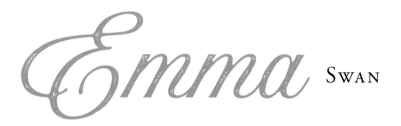

Emma SWAN

Talk about a storied past! Though Emma Swan, played by the American actress Jennifer Morrison, grew up in foster care in Minnesota, she is actually the daughter of Snow White and Prince Charming of Storybrooke, Maine. Now it is up to her ten-year-old son, whom she gave up for adoption as a baby, to return her to Storybrooke, where she can bring back happy storybook endings.

Most of the time, Emma's style in this enchanted environment is modern, with jeans, a leather jacket, and her hair worn loose. When she becomes the Dark One in season five, however, she sports a looped braided bun. It looks intricate and fancy, but it isn't hard to do. I promise!

SKILL LEVEL: Easy
TIME: 10 minutes

MATERIALS NEEDED:

2 small hair elastics

Hair clips

Bobby pins

Extensions (optional)

Silver hair comb (optional)

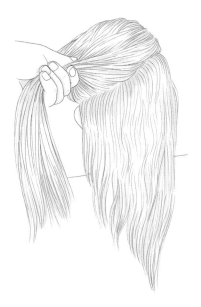

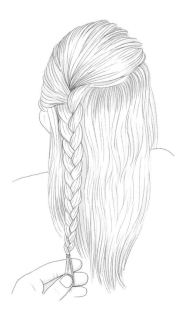

I. Split the hair into two sections, making a diagonal part across the back of the head.

2. English-braid the top section of hair and secure it with a small hair elastic at the end.

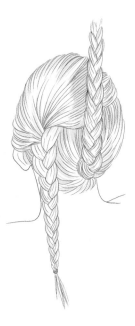

3. English-braid the bottom section of hair to the ends, but direct this braid upward. (If this is difficult, you can try flipping your head upside down in order to braid this section.) Secure the ends of the braid with a small hair elastic.

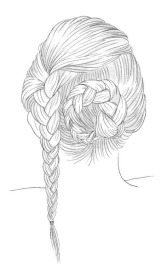

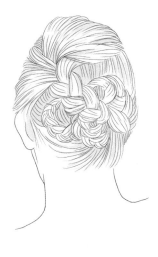

4. Make a circle with the bottom braid at the back of the head, and clip it in place for now; don't pin it down just yet.

5. Now make an interlocking circle with the top braid by passing it through the hole made by the braid circle. Pin both of these braids to the head. Tuck the elastic-tied ends of the braids underneath the circles to hide them.

Hair Tip

If your hair is thin and you want a big bun like Emma's, you can add some clip-in extensions before making the braids. Also, if you wish, add a silver hair comb like the one Emma wears in the Enchanted Forest.

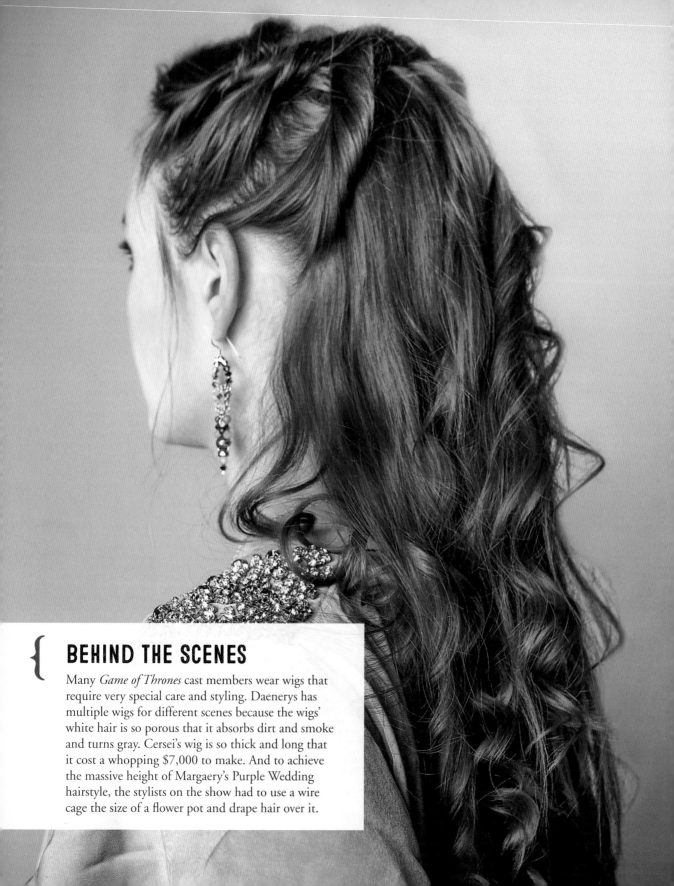

{ BEHIND THE SCENES

Many *Game of Thrones* cast members wear wigs that require very special care and styling. Daenerys has multiple wigs for different scenes because the wigs' white hair is so porous that it absorbs dirt and smoke and turns gray. Cersei's wig is so thick and long that it cost a whopping $7,000 to make. And to achieve the massive height of Margaery's Purple Wedding hairstyle, the stylists on the show had to use a wire cage the size of a flower pot and drape hair over it.

Margaery Tyrell

Played by the English actress Natalie Dormer, Margaery Tyrell is the premier social climber of the Seven Kingdoms. With the goal of being queen—and encroaching upon Cersei Lannister's territory (page 121) in the process—she marries not one, not two, but *three* kings. Her personal style is distinctly graceful, yet seductive, and her hairstyles feature many rope braids and twists, which Sansa Stark (page 129) mimics in season three as she tries to fit in at King's Landing.

SKILL LEVEL: Easy
TIME: 5 minutes

MATERIALS NEEDED:
Bobby pins
Curling iron (optional)

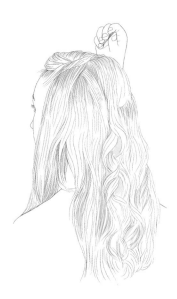

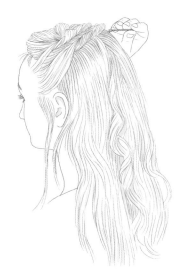

1. Make a center part. Take a small section of hair from above the forehead on one side of the part. Twist this section backward. Gently drape it back to the crown of the head and pin it there, pushing the pins underneath the twist to hide them. Repeat this step on the other side of the head.

2. Pick up another section of hair directly beneath the first one, twist it, and pin it at the crown. Repeat this step on the other side of the head.

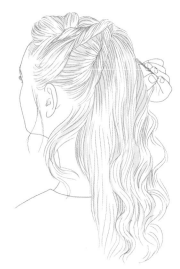

Hair Tip

Curly or wavy hair makes this style more romantic, so if your hair is stick straight, you may want to create soft curls with a curling iron to finish the look.

3. Finally, make one more tier of twists below these, picking up hair from right above and behind the ears.

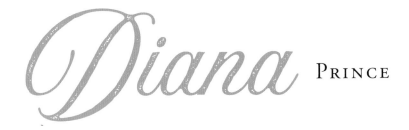

Diana PRINCE

She fights ferociously, inspires truth, wields God-given weapons, and builds a better world—even just talking about Wonder Woman gets you fired up and feeling empowered! Played by the Israeli actress Gal Gadot, this Amazonian princess is training for battle on her home island of Themyscira, when Steve Trevor, an American World War I pilot, crashes nearby and requires her immediate assistance. Her battle-braid style is based on the French fishtail technique, with a slight adjustment to hold it in place.

SKILL LEVEL: Intermediate
TIME: 10 minutes

MATERIALS NEEDED:
1 small or large hair elastic

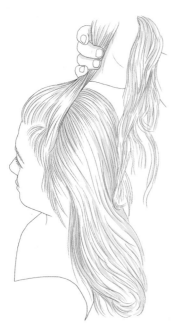

1. Section the hair from the tops of the ears to the top of the head.

2. Start making a French fishtail braid with this hair. Collect more hair from the left side of the head to add into the braid as you do with French-braid styles, but pass it underneath the braid first. Then add it to some hair from the right half of the fishtail braid and bring it over to add it to the inside of the other fishtail strand. Do the same thing with hair from the other side of the head, passing it underneath the braid, adding it to some hair from the left half of the fishtail braid, and bringing it over to add it in to the inside of the other strand. This is just like normal French fishtail braiding, except new hair is passed underneath the braid first before adding it to the braid, unlike a French fishtail where new hair is added directly to the inside of the fishtail strands.

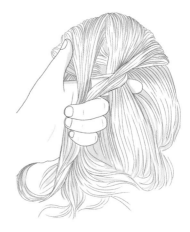

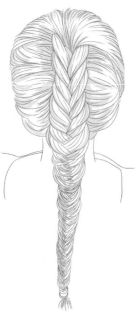

3. Keep forming the fishtail braid like this, passing hair from the opposite side of the head underneath the braid and then adding it in. This gives the braid a downward chevron pattern, but makes it sit on top of the head like a Dutch fishtail braid. It also adds more friction to the style so the braid holds together better. When there's no more hair to add in, finish the braid to the ends as a normal fishtail and secure it with the hair elastic.

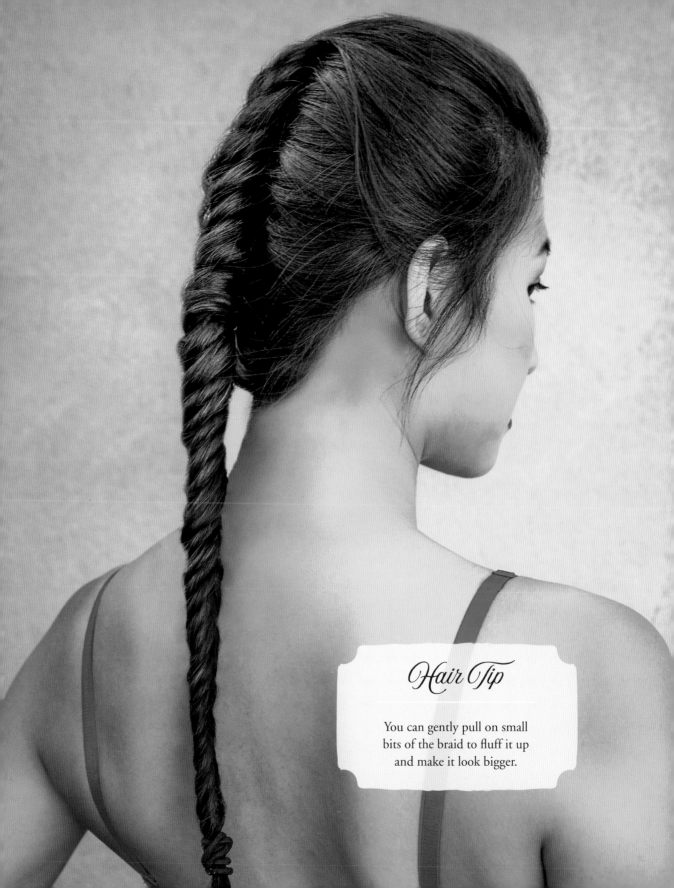

Hair Tip

You can gently pull on small bits of the braid to fluff it up and make it look bigger.

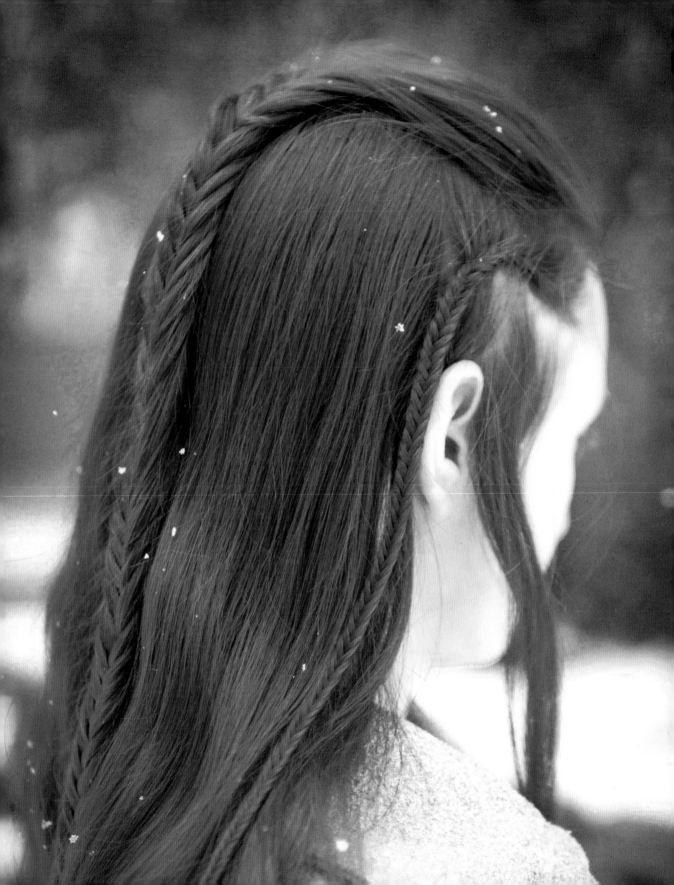

Legolas

Sent as a messenger by his father to the Council of Elrond, Legolas, played by the English actor Orlando Bloom, volunteers to represent the elves as one of the nine members of the Fellowship of the Ring. With his mad archery skills, heightened senses, and strikingly perfect hair, this Prince of the Woodland Realm is an asset on the quest to destroy the One Ring.

Legolas wears this fishtail braid style in all three of *The Lord of the Rings* movies, as well as in *The Hobbit* trilogy.

SKILL LEVEL: Intermediate
TIME: 15 minutes

MATERIALS NEEDED:
1 small hair elastic

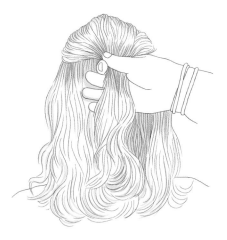

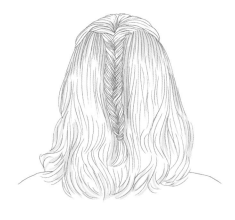

1. Collect all the hair on top of the head into a ponytail at the crown.

2. Fishtail-braid this section of hair all the way to the ends, and secure it with a hair elastic.

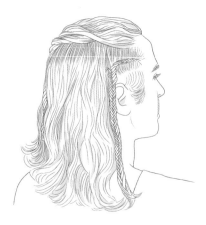

3. Pick up a small section of hair on one side of the head and make a lace fishtail braid. Keep adding in small amounts of hair from the side of the head until you get past the ears, then stop adding in new hair and finish the fishtail braid normally to the ends. Let the ends of these braids hang without securing them, because small braids hold themselves together well. Repeat this step on the other side of the head.

Morgana PENDRAGON

When her magical powers materialize, this good girl, played by the Irish actress Katie McGrath, turns bad. Uther Pendragon, Morgana and King Arthur's father, outlawed magic in Camelot, and those who are caught practicing it may be sentenced to death. Morgana isn't keen to give up her powers so easily, leaving her with little option but to turn against family and friends as she plots to take over the kingdom.

Style-wise, Morgana's fall from grace is reflected in her hair, which becomes increasingly disheveled, but when she is momentarily crowned queen, after she and the sorceress Morgause capture Camelot, she wears this side-braided look.

SKILL LEVEL: Intermediate
TIME: 20 minutes

MATERIALS NEEDED:
Hair clips
4 small hair elastics
1 large hair elastic

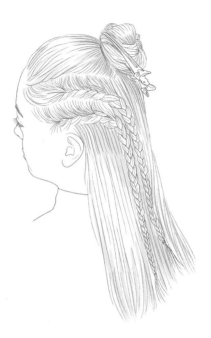

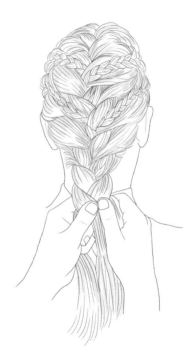

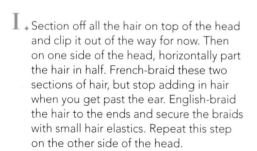

1. Section off all the hair on top of the head and clip it out of the way for now. Then on one side of the head, horizontally part the hair in half. French-braid these two sections of hair, but stop adding in hair when you get past the ear. English-braid the hair to the ends and secure the braids with small hair elastics. Repeat this step on the other side of the head.

2. Take the hair gathered on top of the head, and start French-braiding it down the back. Add in all the hair on the head, as well as the four smaller French braids when you get to them. Finish the French braid to the ends and secure it with the large hair elastic.

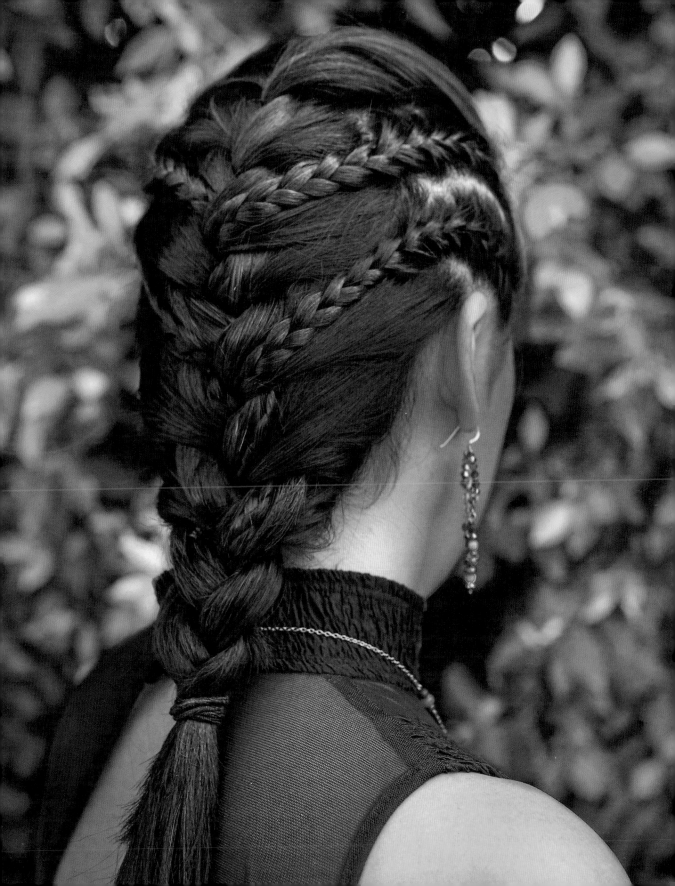

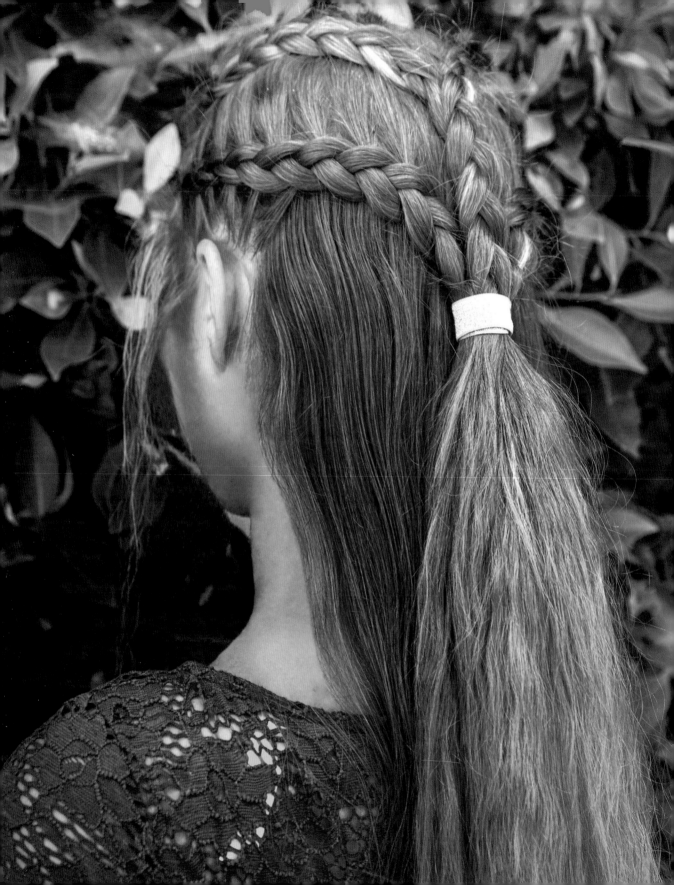

Daenerys Targaryen

The Mother of Dragons, played by English actress Emilia Clarke, has arguably one of the most iconic hairstyles ever shown on-screen. While her look has evolved over many seasons, from girlish waves to tight braided buns and ponytails, Dany almost always wears some sort of tiered braid look, reflecting the importance of braids to Dothraki culture and in turn the importance of being a Khaleesi to her character formation.

Daenerys wears this style in the third and fourth seasons, during the time she is conquering the cities of Slaver's Bay.

SKILL LEVEL: Intermediate
TIME: 15 minutes

MATERIALS NEEDED:

2 small hair elastics

1 large hair elastic

Curling iron (optional)

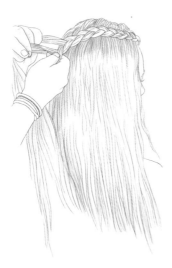

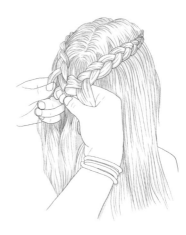

1. Make a center part, and then create a Dutch lace braid that starts at one of the corners of the forehead and goes directly backward. When you reach the crown, stop adding in new hair and braid the hair to the ends. Secure it with an elastic for now. Repeat this step on the other side of the part.

2. Bring the braids together at the crown. Use your fingers to poke holes in between the strands of these braids and line up the three strands from one braid with the three strands from the other braid.

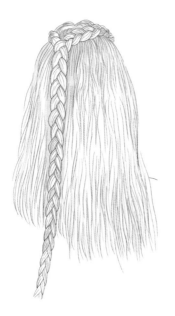

3. Undo the braiding below this point and blend together the strands from the two braids. With these new, larger strands, English-braid the hair to the ends. Again, secure temporarily with an elastic.

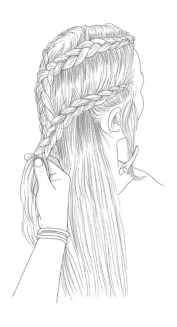

4. Now make a Dutch braid on one side of the head, leaving out a bit of wispy hair around the face. Dutch-braid straight back until you reach the ear, then stop adding in hair to the bottom of the braid and make a Dutch lace braid the rest of the way instead, only adding in hair to the top strands of the braid (the strands closest to the top of the head). Stop adding in new hair when you reach the back of the head and finish the braid to the ends. Repeat this step on the other side of the head.

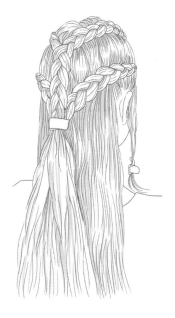

5. At the center of the back of the head, secure these three braids together with the large hair elastic. Release the braiding below this elastic.

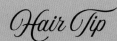

Hair Tip

After finishing the braids, curl the remaining loose hair to look even more like Dany!

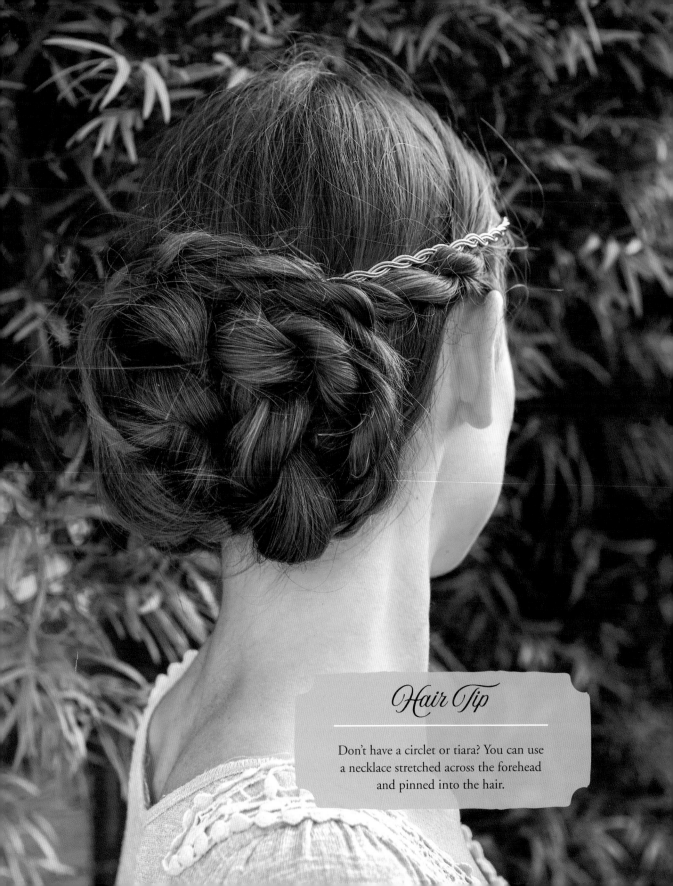

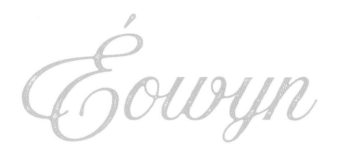

Lady Éowyn of Rohan is one of the few female characters in *The Lord of the Rings* trilogy. Though her storyline varies a little between the books and the movies, in both she is brave and fiercely loyal to her people. She eventually becomes temporary leader of Rohan during Théoden's battle against the army of Isengard and then a warrior when she disguises herself as a man and slays the Witch-king of Angmar at the Battle of the Pelennor Fields.

Played by Australian actress Miranda Otto, Éowyn wears this elegant updo worn during Théodred's funeral, when she sings a lament for the fallen prince.

SKILL LEVEL: Intermediate
TIME: 15 minutes

MATERIALS NEEDED:

Gold circlet or tiara
4 small hair elastics
Bobby pins

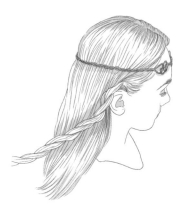

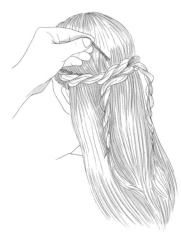

1. Place the gold circlet on the head before you begin braiding. Pick up a section of hair along the front hairline that spans between the center part and the ear. Rope-braid this section of hair to the ends and secure it with a small elastic. Repeat this step on the other side of the head.

2. Cross these rope braids at the back of the head and pin them in place. Let any extra length of braid hang free for now.

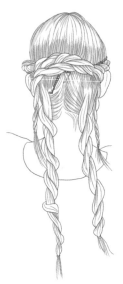

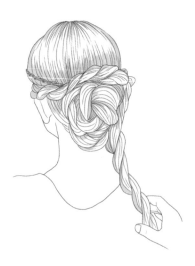

3. Split the remaining hair in half, then rope-braid each half to the ends. Secure these braids with small elastics.

4. Coil up these braids on the back of the head into a vertical elongated shape, pinning as you go. Position the braid buns right next to each other so that there's no gap between them. If you have any extra length in the first pair of braids, wrap it around the braid buns and secure with bobby pins. Make sure to tuck the ends of the braids underneath the bun to hide them.

Tauriel

Introduced for the first time in Peter Jackson's film adaptations of *The Hobbit*, Tauriel, whose name translates to "Daughter of the Forest," is captain of the Mirkwood Elven Guard. Played by the Canadian actress Evangeline Lilly, this skilled warrior and healer fights alongside the elf prince Legolas (page 105), helping to defeat the evil orcs and their chieftain.

Tauriel's look is a great visual representation of her character. The fishtail and rope braids are ethereal elements that other elves incorporate, but hers function to pull the hair backward and keep it out of her face for battle. Further, the lace-braid design on top of her head resembles armor, hinting at her fighting prowess.

SKILL LEVEL: Intermediate
TIME: 20 minutes

MATERIALS NEEDED:

Hair clips
1 or 2 small hair elastics

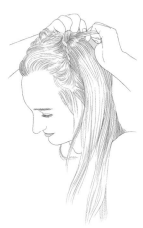

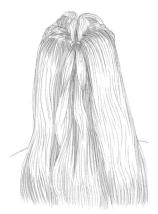

1. Pick out a small section of hair right in front of each of the ears and clip it out of the way. Then make a lace braid on either side of the head that starts just above the ear and ends at the top back of the head. Add in hair to just the upper strands of the lace braid and aim it toward the crown so that it angles upward as you are forming it.

2. Tie together the two braids at the crown with a small hair elastic.

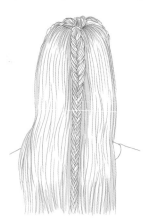

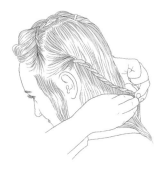

3. Undo any lace braiding below the tie, then make a fishtail braid. Temporarily secure the end with a clip or elastic.

4. Now pick up a small section of hair from right next to where the lace braid started, and rope-braid this section. Repeat this step on the other side of the head.

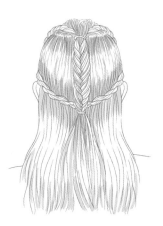

5. Tie these rope braids and the fishtail braid together at the center of the back of the head, then undo any braiding below this tie.

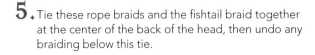

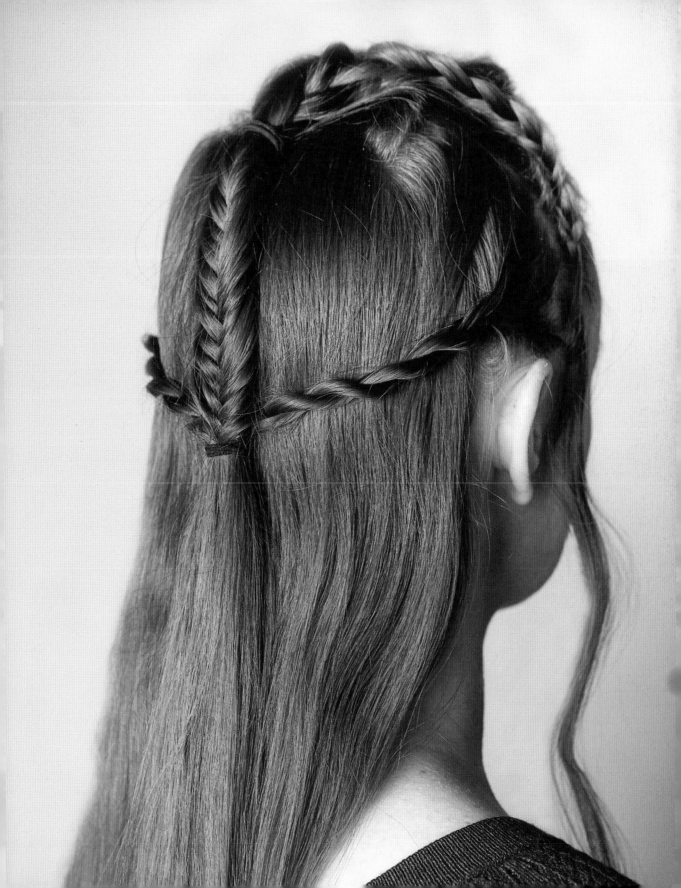

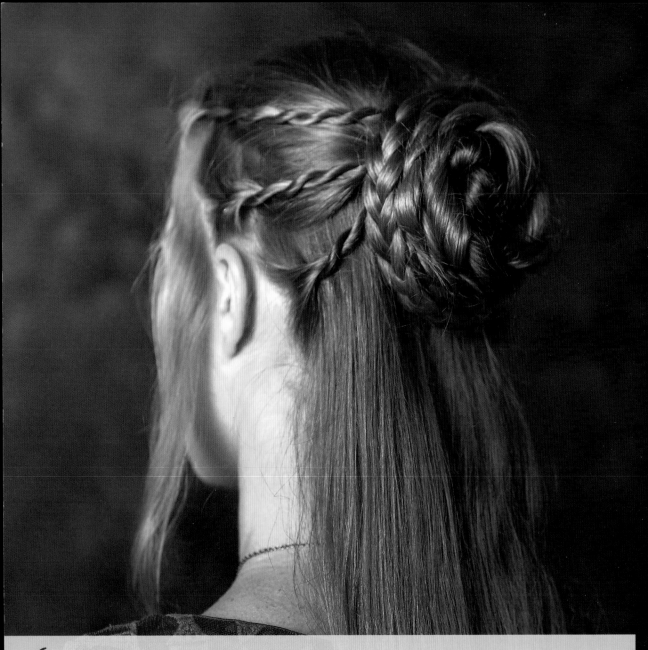

{ BEHIND THE SCENES

Game of Thrones lead stylist Kevin Alexander shared tips about how he creates beautiful and spiraling loose curls on the women in the series. First, he treats the hair with Wella setting products and then wraps it around a Cloud Nine curling wand. After that, the hair is held in position with clips overnight. Differences in hair texture will affect how each head of hair responds to this treatment, but setting lotion and a long setting time will really help pretty much everyone get lasting curls!

Cersei LANNISTER

Skillfully played by the Emmy-nominated English actress Lena Headey, Cersei Lannister is the *Game of Thrones* character everyone loves to hate. Despite showing a tender side toward her children and their father (her handsome brother Jamie), this Queen of the Seven Kingdoms is merciless and vengeful on her quest for the Iron Throne. Sansa Stark (page 129) and Margaery Tyrell (page 99) can attest to this!

The style shown here is from early in the show, when she has a full head of golden locks. The braid bun and rope braid elements are very in fashion with the way high-born women wore their hair in southern Westeros.

SKILL LEVEL: Advanced
TIME: 30 minutes

MATERIALS NEEDED:

8 small hair elastics

Hair clips

Bobby pins

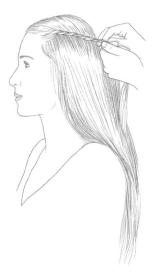

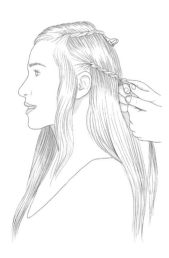

1. Make a center part, then pick up a small amount of hair on either side of the part at the forehead. Rope-braid these sections and secure the ends with small hair elastics.

2. Pick up another small section of hair on each side of the head and rope-braid these as well, securing them with small elastics. Make sure to leave out a bit of hair along the hairline to hang in front of the ears.

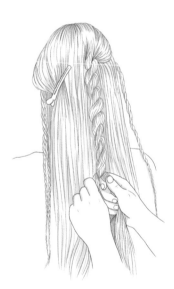

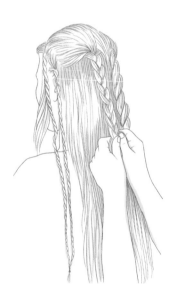

3. Now gather up the hair at the top of the back of the head so that you're holding about half of the remaining free hair. Divide this into left and right halves. Clip the left half out of the way for now, then rope-braid the right half and secure it with a small elastic.

4. English-braid the left half and secure the ends with a small hair elastic.

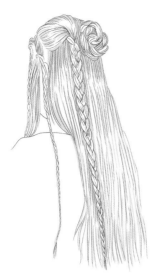

5. Coil up the large rope braid into a bun at the top center of the back of the head, pinning it in place.

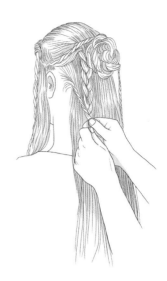

6. Make a third tier of small rope braids, starting behind the ears. Secure them with small elastics.

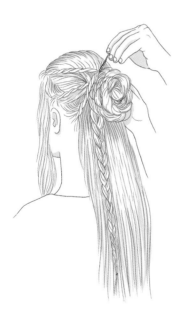

7. Wrap the six small rope braids around the large rope-braid bun, pinning them in place. Make sure to tuck the ends of each braid underneath the bun to hide them.

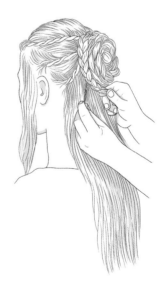

8. Finally, pin the English braid around the bun.

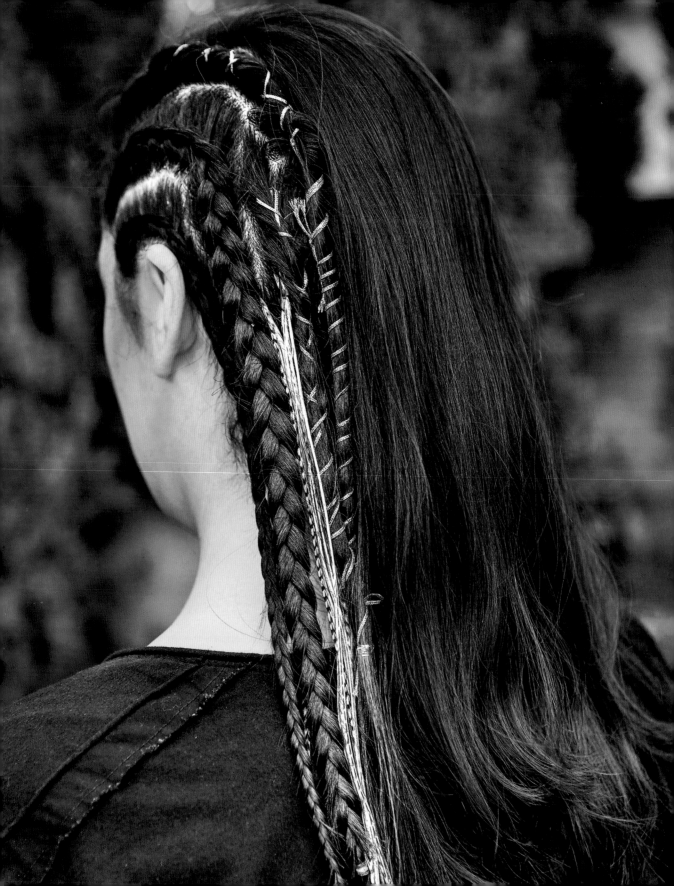

Eretria

Eretria, played by the Spanish actress Ivana Baquero, begins the first season of *The Shannara Chronicles* as a Rover—a nomadic people who sometimes thieved or worked as mercenaries to survive. On her first solo thieving mission, she encounters the half-human/half-elf Wil and the elven princess Amberle, and after a tug-of-war over Elfstones, they team up to protect the Four Worlds from demons escaping from their place of banishment: the ancient tree, Ellcrys.

This style is Eretria's eye-catching side-braid look.

SKILL LEVEL: Advanced
TIME: 30 minutes

MATERIALS NEEDED:

Hair clips

2 small hair elastics

2 small, clear hair elastics

Colorful thread

Blunt needle

Feather extensions

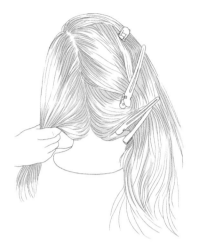 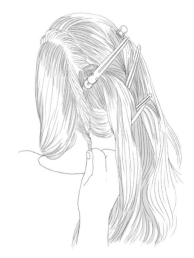

1. Make a C-shaped part from one corner of the forehead down to the neck (as if you were sectioning off hair for a side shave). Clip or tie the larger section of hair out of the way; you won't be using it.

2. Section off a strip of hair on the side of the head that runs two-thirds of the way along the C-shaped part and is about 1 inch (2.5 cm) wide. Tightly twist this section. Clip it up for now so that it doesn't unravel. With the remaining one-third of hair along the part, make a second twist and clip it for now.

Hair Tip

If it's too difficult to keep the twists in step 2 in place, braid this hair into two lace-rope braids instead, so that they hold together better.

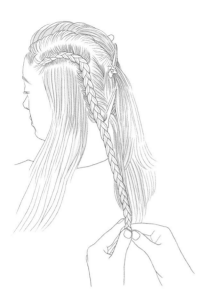

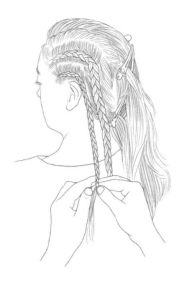

3. Horizontally divide the remaining hair in half. Dutch-braid the top section to the ends and secure it with a small hair elastic.

4. Make another Dutch braid with the remaining hair, and secure it with a small hair elastic.

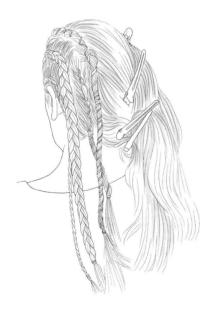

5. With the thread and blunt needle, sew the thread around the first twist all the way to the ends of the hair, twisting the hair as you go. Secure the ends with a small, clear hair elastic to hold it all in place. Now wrap up the second twist with more thread and secure it with another elastic. Lastly, pin some feather extensions underneath the second twist so that they hang among the braids.

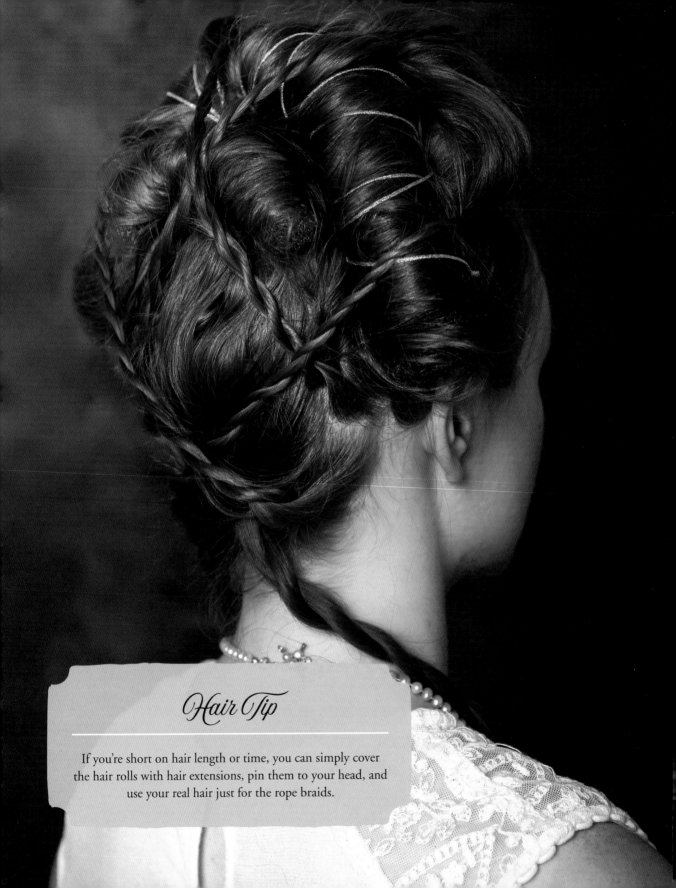

Hair Tip

If you're short on hair length or time, you can simply cover the hair rolls with hair extensions, pin them to your head, and use your real hair just for the rope braids.

GAME OF THRONES

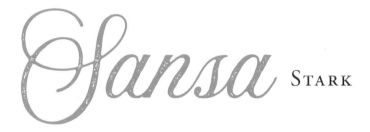

Sansa STARK

Every character in *Game of Thrones* has to figure out a way to survive the dangerous politics of Westeros—or perish. Sansa Stark, played by English actress Sophie Turner, practices the subtle art of blending in, always shifting her look in order to fit into each new environment she encounters. For example, at the very beginning of the show, she wears lace and French braids on top of her head, in the Northern style. Once in King's Landing, however, she adopts this elaborate eighteenth century–inspired padded style common to the Southern ladies.

SKILL LEVEL: Advanced
TIME: 40 minutes

MATERIALS NEEDED:

Hair clips

3 hair rolls

Bobby pins

Comb

Hairspray

Blunt needle and thick white thread

Several small hair elastics

Jeweled hair decoration

Extensions (optional)

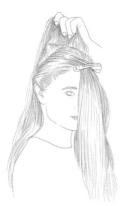

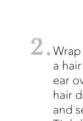

1. Make a section of hair a few inches wide, reaching from ear to ear over the top of the head like a headband. Make another section just like this one directly behind it, wide enough to reach about to the crown of the head. Clip each section for now.

2. Wrap the ends of this second section around a hair roll that is long enough to reach ear to ear over the top of the head. (I'm using foam hair donuts that have been cut into tubes and sewn together to get the correct length.) Tightly roll up this section of hair.

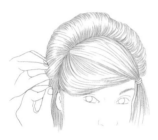

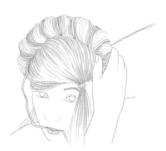

3. Slide the hair outward to cover the entire hair roll, and then pin it down to the head. Gently smooth the hair on the roll with a comb and hairspray.

4. With a blunt needle, sew some thick white thread around this roll.

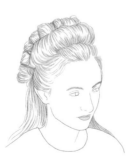

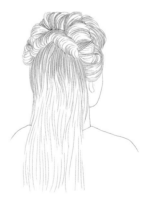

5. Next, roll up the first section by the forehead. This roll should be a little shorter than the first. Again, roll it tight, slide the hair to cover the whole roll, pin it in place, and use a comb and hairspray to make it smooth.

6. For the last roll, pick up a small section at the crown and roll it up. Pin it directly behind the big roll on top of the head.

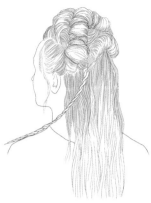

7. Make two rope braids on either side of this small roll.

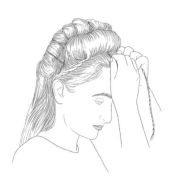

8. Pin these rope braids around the ends of the rolls and in front of the front roll.

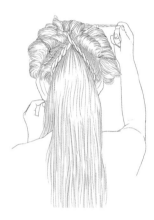

9. Make two more rope braids, one behind each ear. Cross them at the back of the head. Drape them over all the rolls and pin down in front of the first roll.

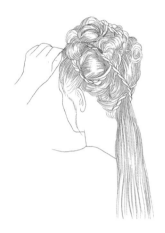

10. Make two more rope braids, this time at the corners of the back hairline. Cross these braids at the back as well, drape over the rolls, and pin in front. If the hair isn't long enough to make the braids reach all the way over the rolls, you can pin them in between the two top rolls or behind the largest roll.

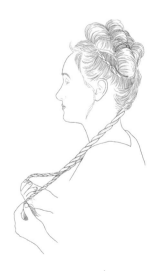

11. Divide the last of the hair in two and cross these sections. Rope-braid each of these sections and let the rope braids hang over each shoulder. Finish the style by placing the jeweled hair decoration in front of the first roll, centered at the top of the head like a small tiara.

131

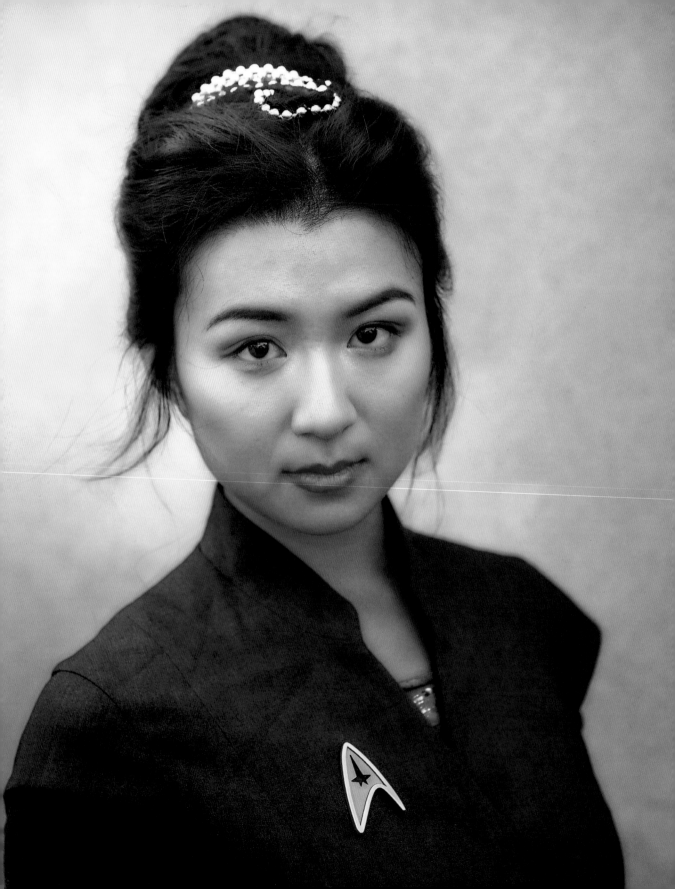

CHAPTER 6

Sci-Fi Heroines

Science fiction is all about the strange and imaginative stories that explore the furthest reaches of possibility. In this chapter, you will learn to make hairstyles from many popular and highly regarded shows and movies that epitomize the sci-fi aesthetic, where outer space and post-apocalyptic wastelands are frequent backdrops for all kinds of heroics. "In a galaxy far, far away," the *Star Wars* trilogy of trilogies (original, prequel, and sequel) features some of the most badass heroines in the history of sci-fi cinema, including **Leia Organa**, **Padmé Amidala**, and **Rey**, as they battle the "dark side" of the Force. *Star Trek: The Next Generation*, which aired from 1987 to 1994, follows the crew of the USS *Enterprise* (NCC-1701-D), including the half-Betazoid lieutenant commander **Deanna Troi**, as they "boldly go where no one has gone before." Back on Earth, a Wild West–themed amusement park is the setting of *Westworld*, where humans pay big bucks to interact with android hosts such as the beautiful Mariposa Saloon madam **Maeve Millay**. Based on the YA book series by Kass Morgan, *The 100* tracks the journey of one hundred teenage prisoners, including **Octavia Blake**, who are packed off to post-apocalyptic planet Earth to get a sense of its (in)habitability. Youths are also sacrificed—in this case, fighting to their deaths—in *The Hunger Games* series, based on the bestselling YA book trilogy by Suzanne Collins. Among them is **Katniss Everdeen**, whose heroics make her an instant celebrity, and with assistance from the documentary filmmaker **Cressida**, a spokeswoman for the rebellion against the Capitol. Moving from a dystopia to a galaxy with a jammin' 1970s soundtrack, *Guardians of the Galaxy* follows a ragtag group of misfits, including the green-skinned Zen-Whoberin assassin **Gamora**, who sets out to save the universe.

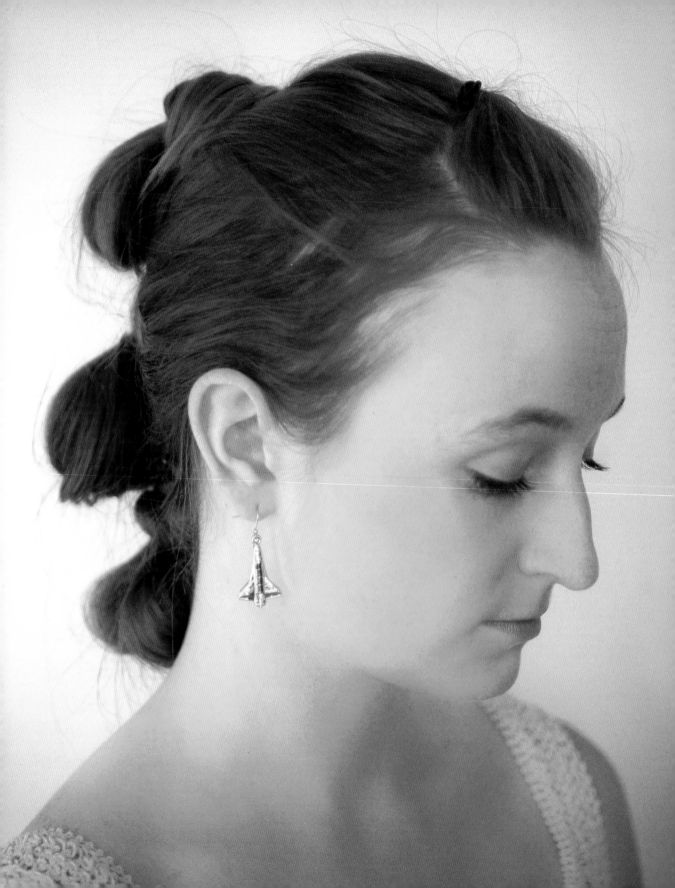

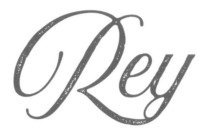

The protagonist of the *Star Wars* sequel trilogy, Rey, played by the English actress Daisy Ridley, is strong, independent, and Force-sensitive. Growing up as an orphan on the desert planet Jakku, Rey supports herself by scavenging parts from old spaceships and tinkering with them. After she escapes from Jakku by piloting the *Millennium Falcon*, she is thrust into a much larger conflict between the Resistance, led by General Leia Organa (page 145), and the sinister First Order.

Rey's hairstyle in these movies is easy to recreate and ideal for anyone whose hair is not quite long enough for more elaborate braided styles.

SKILL LEVEL: Easy
TIME: 5 minutes

MATERIALS NEEDED:

4 small hair elastics

Bobby pins

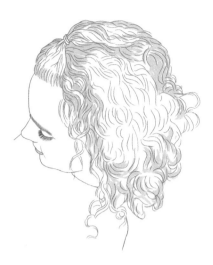

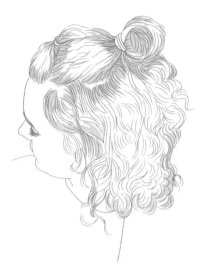

1. Gather the hair at the forehead into a little ponytail and secure it with a small hair elastic. If you have bangs, include this hair in the ponytail.

2. Now gather the hair on top of the head into a ponytail. On the last loop of securing the hair elastic, don't pull the hair all the way through. Leave the ponytail as a club instead. To deal with the remaining tail of hair, wrap it around the ponytail holder and pin it in place.

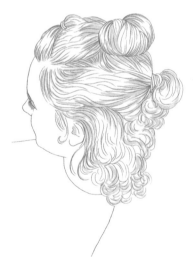

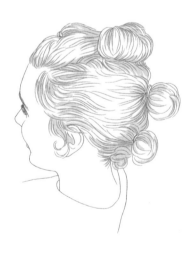

3. With half of the remaining hair, form a second club right below the first one, finishing it as in step 2.

4. Form a third club in the same way with the remaining hair.

Gamora

This alien and former assassin is ready to make amends. Gamora, played by American actress Zoe Saldana, was originally a cold-blooded killer raised to be the ultimate weapon by the evil Thanos. To exact her revenge on Thanos for killing her family and making her this way, she teams up with the rest of the Guardians of the Galaxy in their quest to destroy the fanatical supervillain Ronan.

Being a badass warrior, Gamora doesn't have time for an elaborate hairstyle, so this simple style is great for those who want to add just a bit of attitude to their everyday look.

SKILL LEVEL: Easy
TIME: 5 minutes

MATERIALS NEEDED:
Hairspray or texture spray
2 small hair elastics
Hair beads

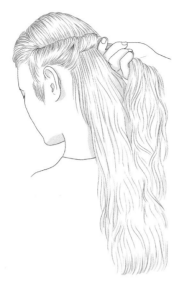

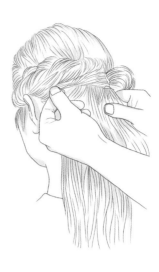

1. Grab a large section of hair from either side of the head. Spray each section with hairspray or texture spray to give the hair more grip. Then twist these sections backward and secure with a small hair elastic at the back of the head.

2. Gently tug on small bits of hair in the twists to fluff them out.

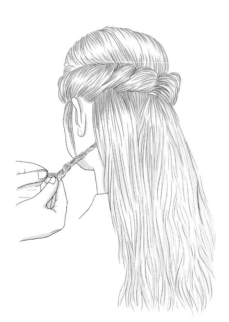

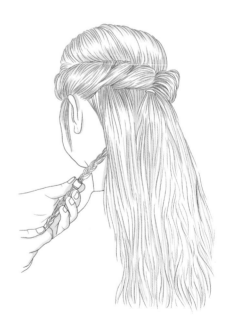

3. On one side of the head, pick up a small section of hair from the lower back hairline. English-braid this hair to the ends and secure with a small hair elastic.

4. Add a couple of hair beads along the length of the braid.

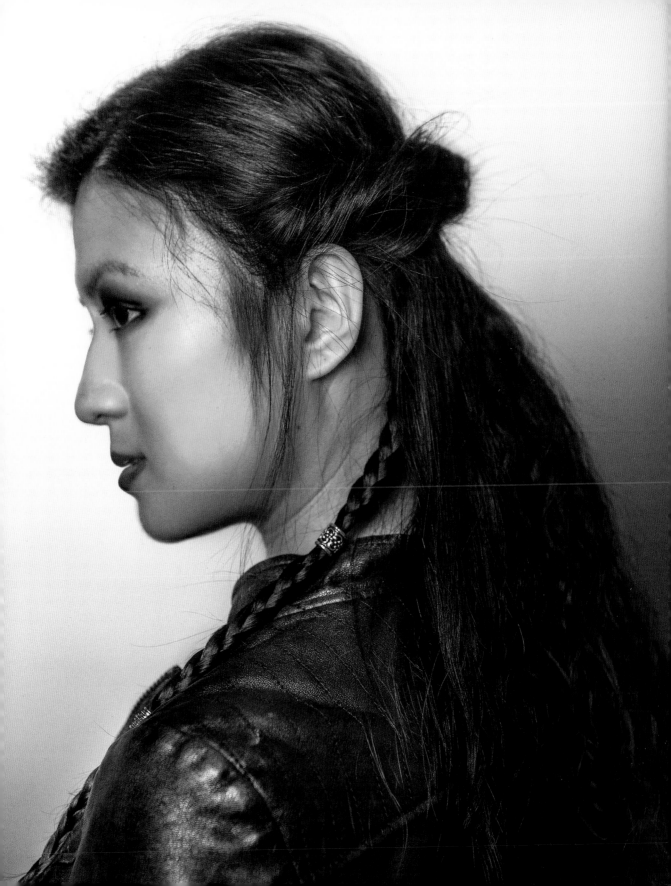

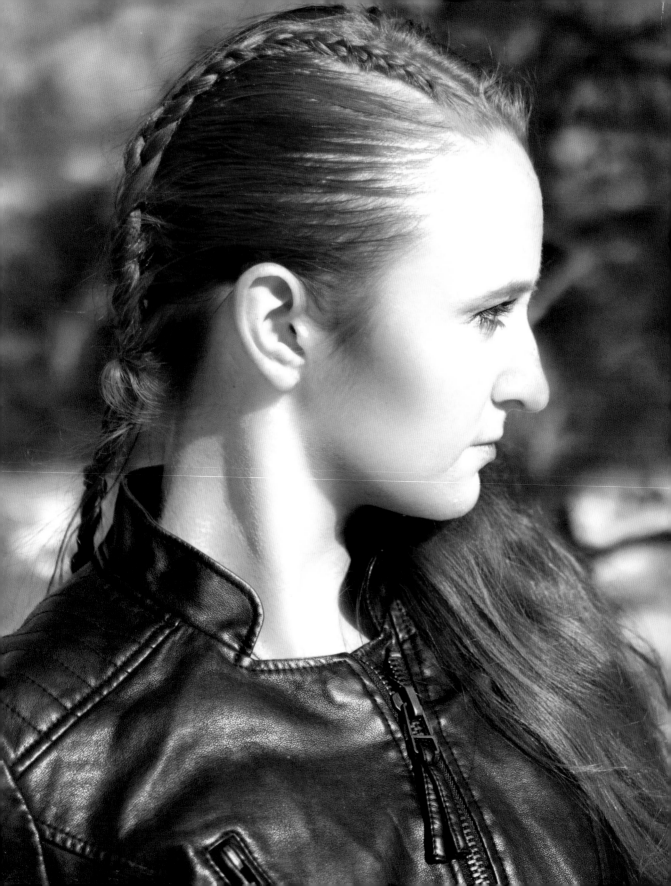

Inspired by

THE HUNGER GAMES: MOCKINGJAY

Cressida

Played by English actress Natalie Dormer, Cressida joins Katniss and the rebellion in the third *The Hunger Games* movie. Her charge is to film the atrocities committed by Capitol forces in the poorer districts in order to erode President Snow's popular support. Cressida rocks a completely side-shaven style, with a little French braid running along the edge of the remaining hair, but you can still approximate her look without taking an electric clipper to one side of your head.

SKILL LEVEL: Intermediate
TIME: 10 minutes

MATERIALS NEEDED:
Rattail comb
Hair clips (optional)
Pomade (optional)
1 small hair elastic

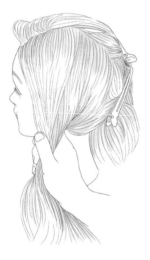

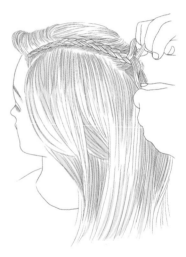

1. Make a part with the pointy end of the comb that starts on the left side of the forehead, runs to the back of the head, continues down the back, and ends at the neck. Clip or tie the larger section of hair out of the way.

2. Make a thin Dutch braid, about ½ inch (13 mm) wide, along the part with hair from the smaller section. Keep braiding until you reach the back of the head.

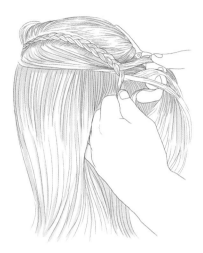

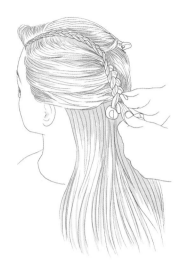

3. Start adding in very small horizontal sections of hair to the Dutch braid from the side of the head. Pull these sections tightly into the braid to hold the hair completely flat against the head, using pomade or the comb, if needed, to smooth the hair against the scalp.

4. Keep weaving these new hair sections into the left strand of the Dutch braid as you form it down the back of the head; make sure you're adding a little bit of hair to the right strand as well so that the braid stays anchored in place next to the part.

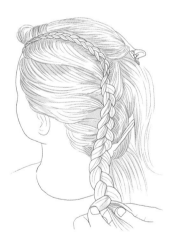

5. When there's no more hair to add into the braid from the side of the head, finish the braid to the ends. Secure it with a small hair elastic.

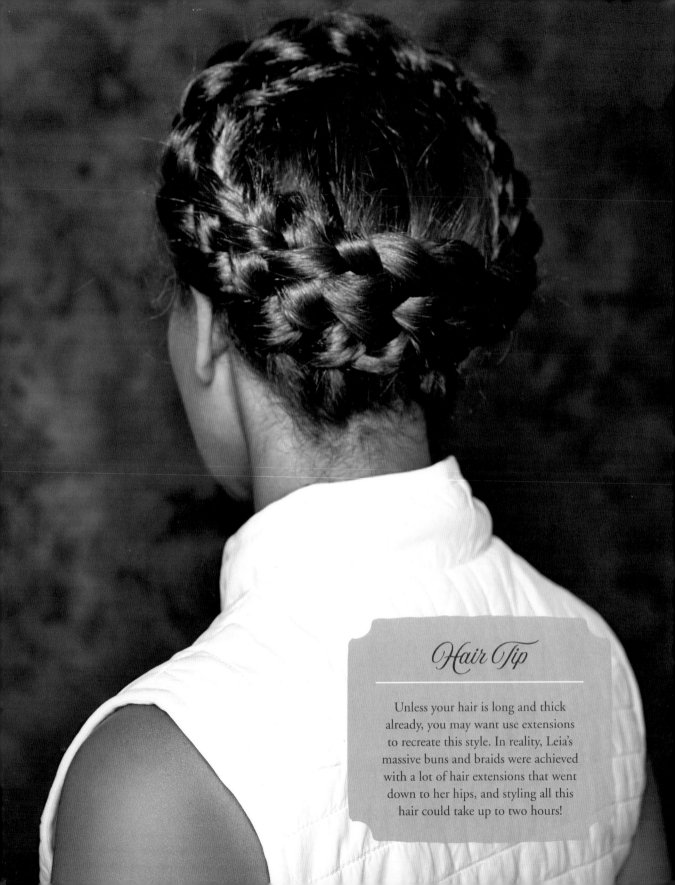

Hair Tip

Unless your hair is long and thick already, you may want use extensions to recreate this style. In reality, Leia's massive buns and braids were achieved with a lot of hair extensions that went down to her hips, and styling all this hair could take up to two hours!

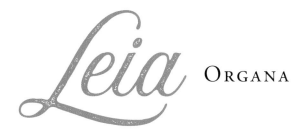 ## Organa

Leia may be only a princess in *Star Wars*, but she is the undisputed queen of sci-fi hairstyles! This 4-foot-11 badass babe, played by the American legend Carrie Fisher, appears in both the original trilogy (as a spy for the Rebel Alliance) and the sequel trilogy (as the general of the Resistance). Raised by Senator Bail and Queen Breha Organa on the planet of Alderaan, she fights alongside her twin brother, Luke Skywalker, and her smuggler-turned-husband, Han Solo, using Force sensitivity to defeat the Galactic Empire and destroy the cataclysmic Death Star.

Leia has many iconic hairstyles through the series, but this is perhaps one of the most wearable and practical.

SKILL LEVEL: Intermediate
TIME: 15 minutes

MATERIALS NEEDED:

2 small hair elastics

Bobby pins

Extensions (optional)

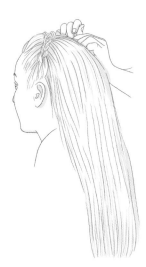

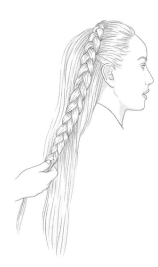

I. Starting at one ear, make a Dutch lace braid that goes over the top and down the other side of the head, like a headband. Incorporate hair from the forehead into one side of this braid.

2. When you reach the other ear, stop adding in new hair, English-braid it to the ends, and secure with a small hair elastic.

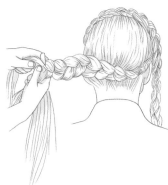

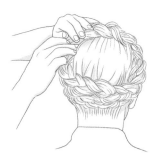

3. With the remaining hair, make a Dutch lace braid across the lower back of the head. Start directly behind the ear where you ended the first braid, and form this braid in the opposite direction. When there's no more hair to add in, English-braid it to the ends and secure with a small hair elastic.

4. Pin both braids along each other into a circular shape. When you get to the ends of the braids, tuck the tails underneath the circle to hide them, then pin them in place.

{ BEHIND THE SCENES

In interviews and books, Carrie Fisher suggested that she was not the biggest fan of her hairdos—the iconic hair donuts were supposedly heavy and painful, and she referred to her updo in *The Force Awakens* as "the baboon butt."

Maeve MILLAY

As an android brothel madam in the Westworld theme park, Maeve, played by the African-English actress Thandie Newton, is the first host to become self-aware. The cunning robot then repeatedly commits suicide so she can return to Livestock Management—not only so she can learn more about the system controlling her, but also to remember her past.

This hairstyle is the look she wears while in full madam getup in the Mariposa Saloon.

SKILL LEVEL: Intermediate

TIME: 15 minutes

MATERIALS NEEDED:

1 large hair elastic	Bobby pins
Hair donut	Feather or flower hair accessory
2 small hair elastics	Extensions (optional)

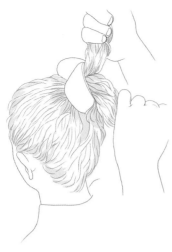

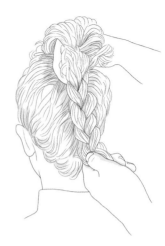

1. Tie all the hair into a very high ponytail with a large hair elastic. Fit the hair donut over the ponytail, then vertically split the ponytail in half.

2. English-braid both halves of the ponytail to the ends and secure with small hair elastics.

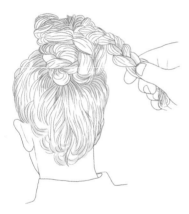

3. Pin one of these braids into a circle on top of the hair donut. Pin the bottom braid around the outside of the donut. With both of these braids pinned, the donut should be completely hidden and the style should look like a large braid bun. Finish with a feather or flower hair accessory attached to the back of the bun.

Hair Tip

Short or fine hair? Make a normal bun with all your hair, and then pin some braids made out of hair extensions around the bun.

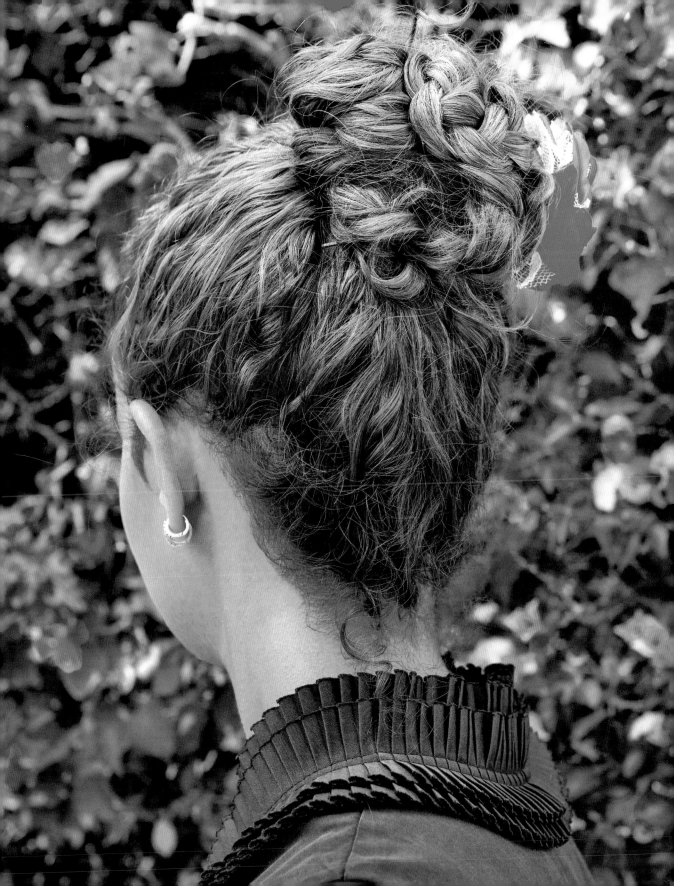

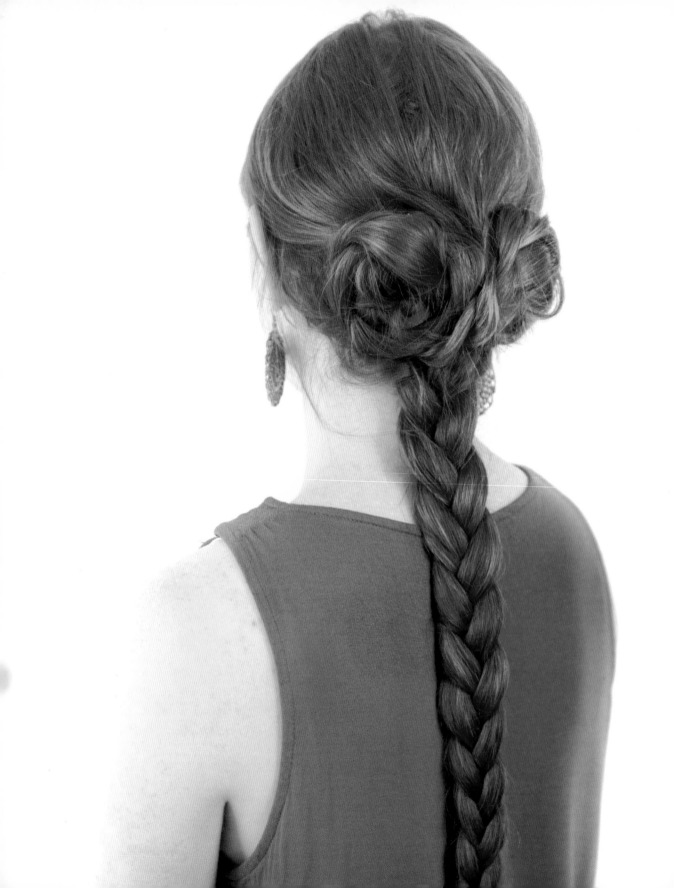

STAR WARS: REVENGE OF THE SITH

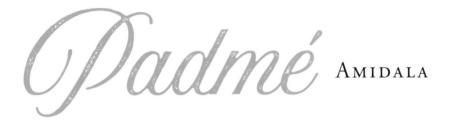 AMIDALA

The protagonist in the prequel trilogy, Padmé Amidala Naberrie, played by the Israeli-American actress Natalie Portman, is elected Queen of Naboo when she is just fourteen years old. Later on, after her reign, she becomes a member of the Galactic Senate and continues her fight for peace and democracy. Perhaps her greatest gift to the galaxy, however, is the birth of twins Luke Skywalker and Princess Leia Organa (page 145), following her covert marriage to the Jedi-turned–Sith Lord Anakin Skywalker (aka Darth Vader).

Padmé wears this hairstyle on Mustafar during her last-ditch effort to persuade Anakin to turn away from the dark side.

SKILL LEVEL: Intermediate
TIME: 10 minutes

MATERIALS NEEDED:

Hair clips

3 small hair elastics

Bobby pins

Extensions (optional)

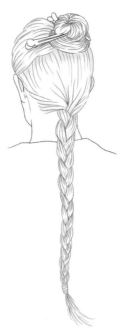

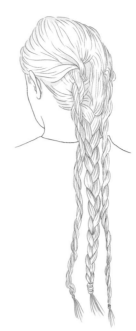

1. Horizontally divide the hair in half. Clip up the top half for now. English-braid the lower half and secure it with a small hair elastic.

2. Take down the hair you clipped up and vertically divide it in half. Rope-braid each half of hair and secure it with small hair elastics.

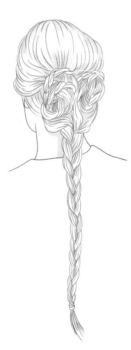

3. Pin these rope braids into circular buns at the top of the English braid. Make sure the buns are touching each other.

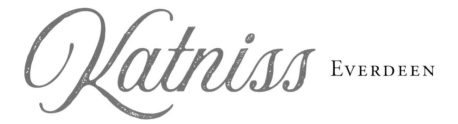

Katniss Everdeen

When Primrose Everdeen is chosen to represent District 12 as its female tribute in the 74th Hunger Games, her older sister, Katniss, volunteers to go in her place. Katniss, played by the American actress Jennifer Lawrence, only ever intended to save her sister, but she ends up winning the Hunger Games and becoming the symbol of hope in a rebellion that erupts throughout the districts.

This hairstyle is the side-braid look Katniss wears in the third movie, when she has become the Mockingjay and is set to battle against the Capitol's forces.

SKILL LEVEL: Intermediate
TIME: 15 minutes

MATERIALS NEEDED:

1 or 2 small hair elastics

Hair clips

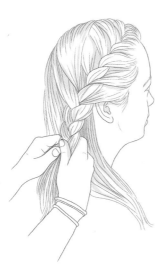

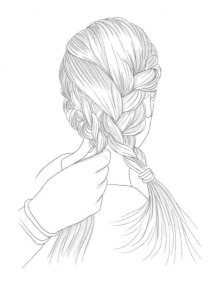

I. Make a French braid along one side of the head, leaving out any bangs. Keep this braid along just the side of the head, adding in no more than half the hair. Stop braiding once you reach the lower back of the head and secure the braid with a small hair elastic or clip for now.

2. Start another French braid on the other side of the head. Form this one along that side, and then continue along the lower back of the head so that it ends next to the first one.

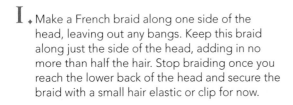

{ BEHIND THE SCENES

In *The Hunger Games*, hairstyling should be an afterthought for those living in the poorer communities outside of the Capitol, but the movie hairstylists had to put in quite a bit of effort to achieve Katniss's look. In the first two movies, her messy Dutch braid was achieved by curling the hair at the roots to give it texture and volume, and then twisting pieces of hair before adding them to the braid. In *Mockingjay*, Jennifer Lawrence had to wear a full wig because her own hair wasn't dark or long enough.

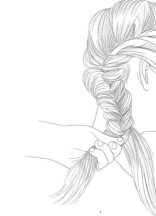

3. Untie the ends of the first braid and blend them with the ends of the second braid. Fishtail-braid this hair to the ends and secure with a hair elastic.

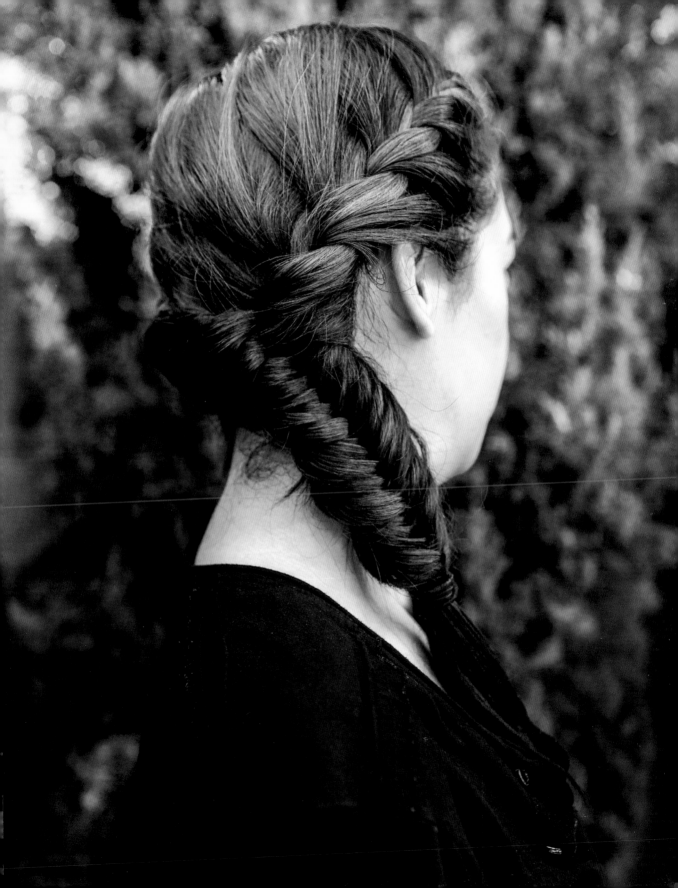

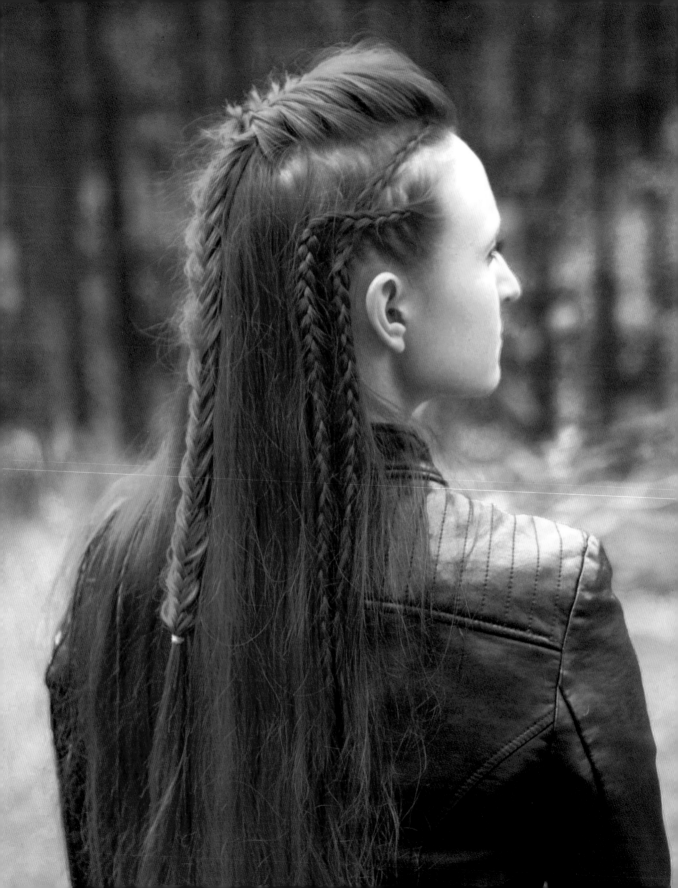

Octavia Blake

Born as an illegal second child on the space station *The Ark*, Octavia, played by the Canadian actress Marie Avgeropoulos, grew up always having to stay hidden. After she is found and imprisoned, she is chosen to accompany the other teens sent to Earth's nuclear wasteland, where she demonstrates a natural ferocity and ultimately bonds with the native Grounder warriors.

Octavia dons this braided style after she has joined the Grounders.

SKILL LEVEL: Advanced
TIME: 30 minutes

MATERIALS NEEDED:

Hair clips
5 small hair elastics

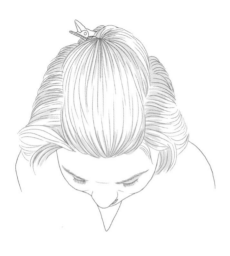

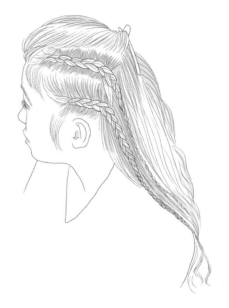

I. Section off the hair on top of the head and clip it out of the way for now.

2. On one side of the head, horizontally divide the hair in half. Dutch-braid the top section of hair until you reach the back of the head, then English-braid it to the ends and secure it with a small hair elastic. Make another Dutch braid below this one with the remaining hair, finishing it with an English braid and securing it with a small hair elastic.

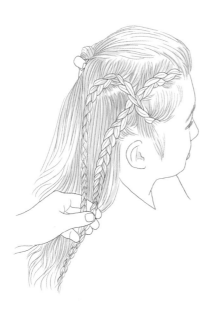

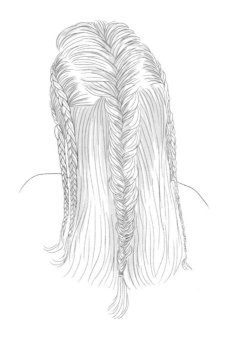

3. On the other side of the head, horizontally divide the hair in half. Dutch-braid the top section, but stop braiding about halfway to the back of the head. Clip up the rest of the hair from this top section, then finish the Dutch braid with hair from the lower half. Start the second Dutch braid below the first one with the remaining lower half of hair. When you get halfway to the back of the head, start braiding in the hair in the remaining top section of hair that you clipped out of the way. This makes the braids cross in the middle. English-braid each of them to the ends and secure with small hair elastics.

4. Make a French fishtail braid with the section of hair on top of the head. Stop adding in hair when you reach the crown, then finish the braid to the ends as a normal fishtail. Secure with a small hair elastic. Fluff the braid to give it more volume and messiness.

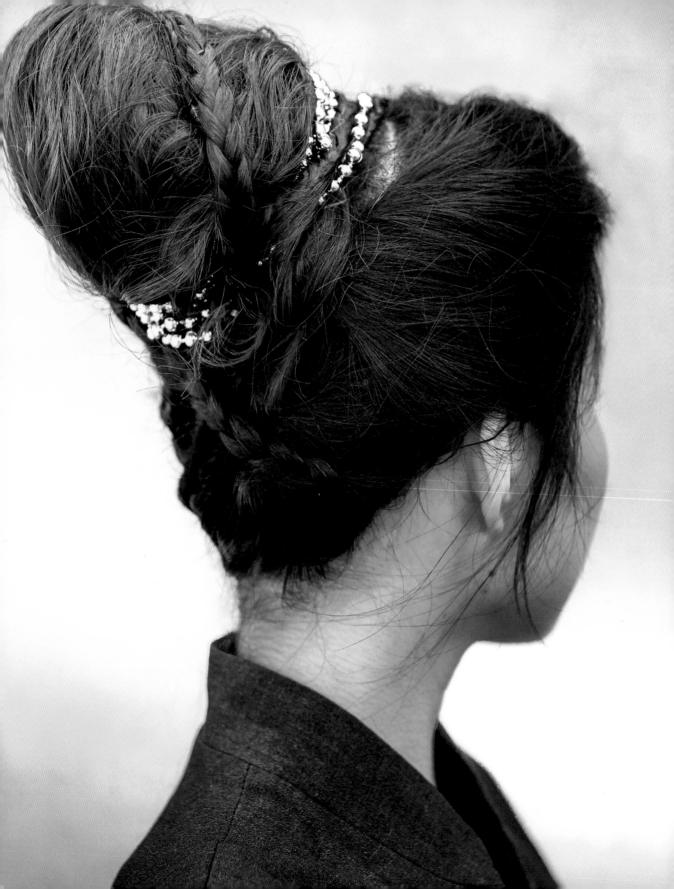

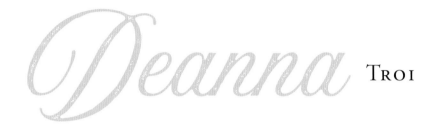

Deanna Troi

USS *Enterprise* lieutenant commander and counselor Deanna Troi, played by the English actress Marina Sirtis, is a natural empath, which comes in handy when the crew comes into contact with other species. Being half Betazoid lends her extrasensory abilities as well. As a half-human lie detector, her insight proves invaluable in many tense encounters and leads her to discover that an alien force invaded the minds of crew members as they transported two enemy alien species—the Anticans and the Selay—to the planet Parliament.

This extravagant bun-and-braids style appears throughout season one. I have no idea who on the ship was willing to style her hair like this every day, but we're going to attempt it now!

SKILL LEVEL: Advanced
TIME: 40 minutes

MATERIALS NEEDED:

1 large hair elastic

2 hair donuts

Bobby pins

Hairspray

4 small hair elastics

2 strings of beads, each one about as long as the hair

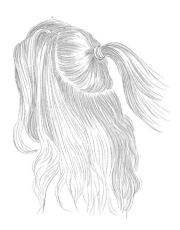

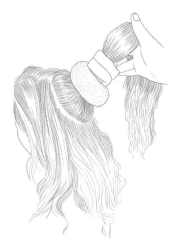

I. Gather a circle of hair at the crown (about half the hair), and tie it into a high ponytail with a large hair elastic.

2. Fit two hair donuts over the ponytail.

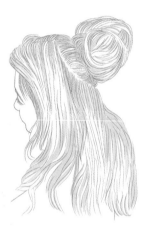

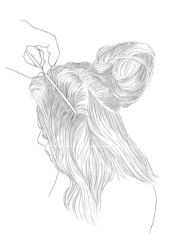

3. With pins and hairspray, smooth the hair from the ponytail around the donuts to completely cover them.

4. Brush forward and tease both the hair in front of the circular ponytail section and the hair on the sides of the head.

Hair Tip

If your hair isn't long enough for these braids to reach very far, braid some small sections of loose hair extensions and pin these to the head instead.

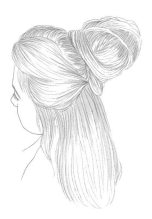

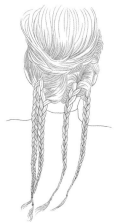

5. Now smooth the teased hair back toward the bun. Pin it against the bun and further smooth and spray the hair around the bun to keep the donuts covered.

6. Divide the remaining hair at the back of the head into four equal sections. English-braid each section, directing the braids upward. Secure the braids with small hair elastics.

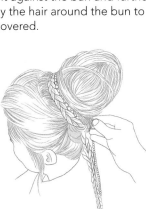

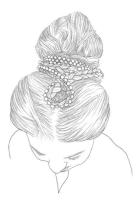

7. Line up a string of beads with one of the braids, and pin both of these around the base of the bun.

8. Line up another string of beads with another braid, and drape it toward the front of the head. Make a loop with this braid and bead string, securing it with pins on top of the center part, near the forehead. Pin the rest of the braid tail and beads around the base of the bun.

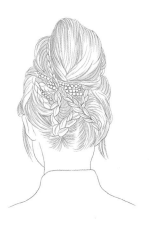

9. Cross the remaining two braids at the back of the head. Spiral them upward around the bun, pinning them in place. Tuck the ends down into the donut hole at the top of the bun.

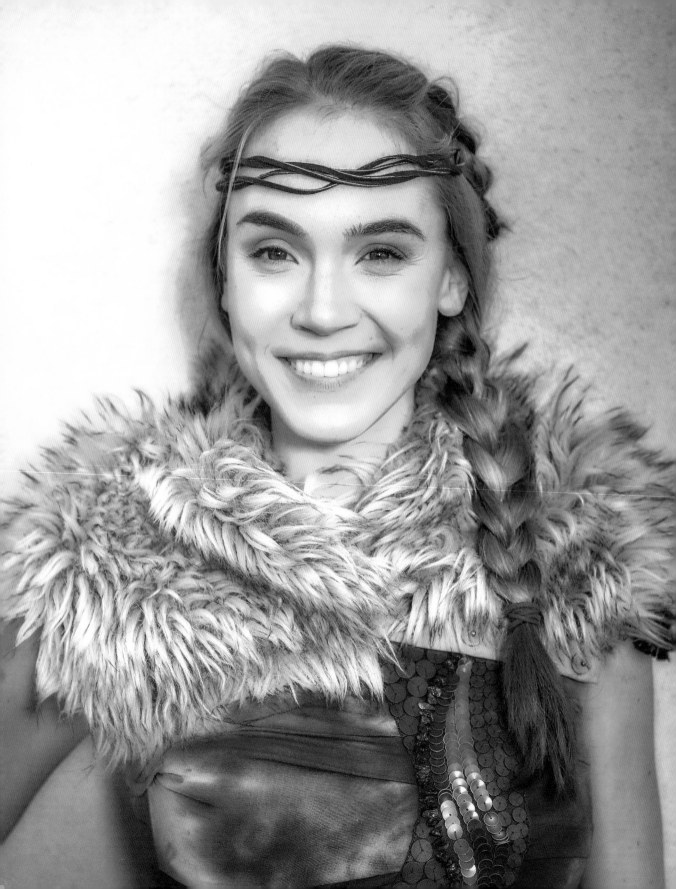

CHAPTER 7

Animated Adventurists

In this chapter, we will leave the land of "real hair" entirely and recreate styles from the animated television series *Sailor Moon* and *Avatar: The Last Airbender*, the animated movie series *How to Train Your Dragon*, and the video game franchises *The Legend of Zelda*, *Assassin's Creed*, *Final Fantasy*, and *Horizon Zero Dawn*. The Japanese anime series *Sailor Moon,* which originally aired in Japan from 1992 to 1997, follows **Usagi Tsukino** (aka Sailor Moon) and the other Sailor Senshi (Mercury, Mars, Jupiter, and Venus) as they defend Earth from evil. In the thirteenth installment of Nintendo's three-decade-old *Legend of Zelda* series, Hyrule crown princess **Zelda** makes the ultimate sacrifice in order to rescue her kingdom from the Twilight. In the Emmy-nominated *Avatar: The Last Airbender*, **Katara** teaches the protagonist Aang the art of Waterbending as they prepare to invade the Fire Nation and restore peace to all nations. **Astrid Hofferson** and her Black Nadder dragon Stormfly are a force to be reckoned with in DreamWorks' *How to Train Your Dragon* series. In the latest of Square Enix's fifteen *Final Fantasy* games, Tenebrae princess **Lunafreya Nox Fleuret** is instrumental in saving the world from a plague of darkness. Ubisoft's *Assassin's Creed Syndicate* takes the age-old fight between the Assassins and the Templars to the streets of Victorian London, where **Evie Frye** and her twin brother attempt to outfox the Blighters. Finally, in *Horizon Zero Dawn*, warrior and outcast **Aloy** is called to save the world, including the people who shunned her, from corrupted machines.

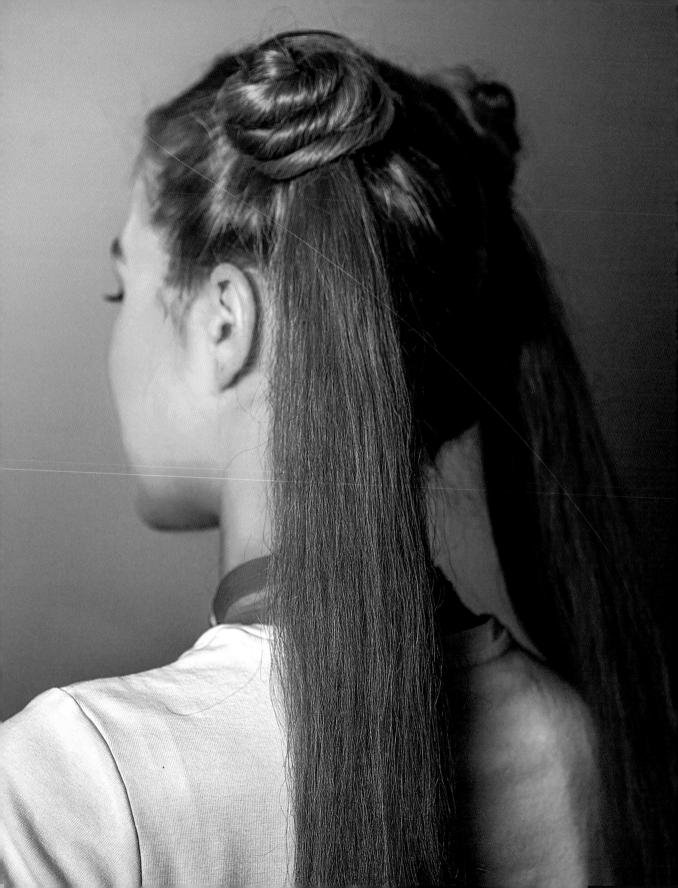

Usagi TSUKINO

When this sailor-suited teen rescues a black cat with a crescent moon on its forehead, she doesn't realize that she will be enlisted to save Earth from the Dark Enemy. After a magic brooch transforms her into Sailor Moon, she joins forces with the Sailor Senshi and Tuxedo Mask, fighting the villainous Queen Beryl, Dead Moon Circus, and countless other antagonists as they seek out the legendary Silver Crystal.

Because anime stories are often hand-drawn, the characters have relatively simple hairstyles, so this style is quite easy to recreate with real hair. Lucky us!

SKILL LEVEL: Easy
TIME: 5 minutes

MATERIALS NEEDED:
2 large hair elastics
Bobby pins

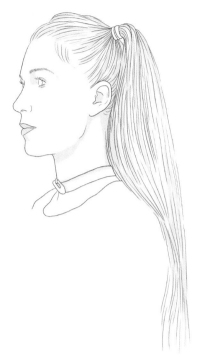

1. Make a center part and vertically divide the hair in half. Tie each half into a high ponytail and secure each with a large hair elastic.

2. Vertically divide the hair of each ponytail in half.

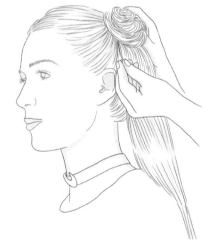

3. Coil half of the hair in each ponytail into a bun on top of the other half and pin it in place. Let the remaining half of the hair hang free.

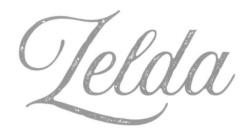

In *The Legend of Zelda: Twilight Princess*, Zelda's kingdom of Hyrule has been taken over by the King of Twilight, and all the inhabitants have turned into wandering spirits. To help save the world, she recruits Link from Ordon Village to revive the Light Spirits and defeat the evil king. Then she does the ultimate selfless act, sacrificing her life and power in order to revive the Twilight creature Midna, who is helping Link on his quest.

SKILL LEVEL: Easy
TIME: 15 minutes

MATERIALS NEEDED:

Hair clips
2 small hair elastics
1 large hair elastic
2 small, clear hair elastics
Thread, about twice as long as the hair
Tiara

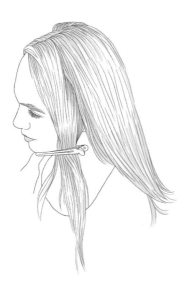

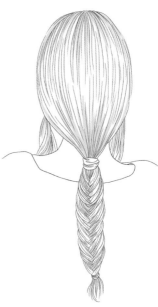

I. Make a center part, then pick out two small sections of hair on either side of the face. Clip these out of the way for now.

2. Now tie the rest of the hair into a loose and low ponytail. Fishtail-braid the hair below this tie, and secure it with a small hair elastic.

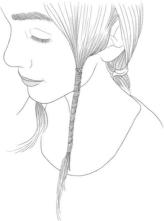

3. Wrap the sections of hair in front of the ears with thread (see Hair Tip). Place the tiara on the head to finish the look.

Hair Tip

It can be difficult to get thread to stay on slippery hair. To keep it in place, use clear hair elastics at the top and bottom of the hair section, wrap the thread around the hair between these elastics, and then tuck the ends of the thread into these elastics.

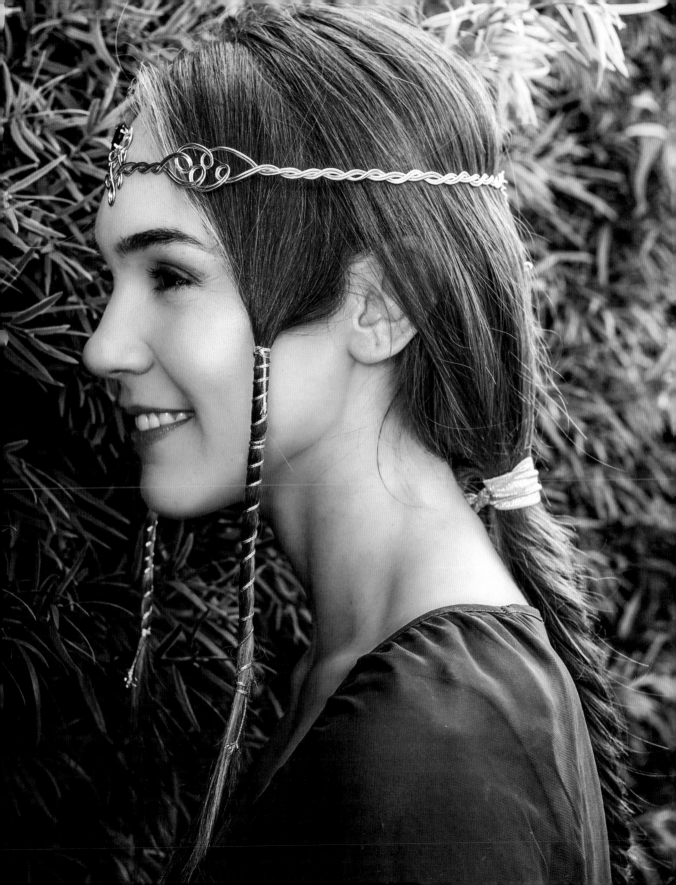

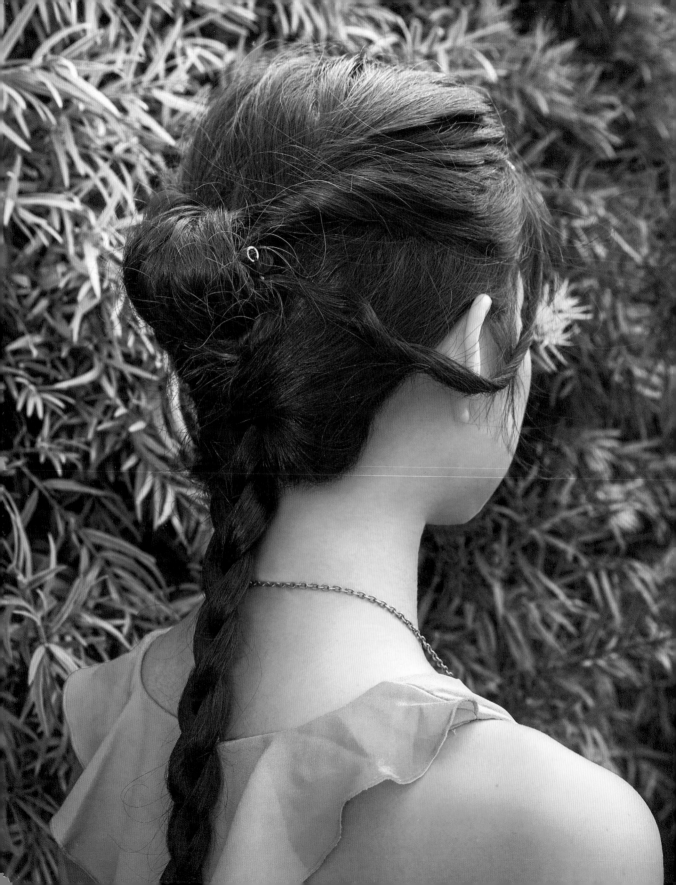

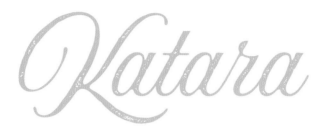

Teenaged Katara and her brother, Sokka, members of the Southern Water Tribe, inadvertently discover a young boy named Aang frozen in a block of ice. When they learn that he is the lost Avatar, they journey out into the wider world to help Aang master all the element-bending arts and eventually defeat tyrant Firelord Ozai.

For much of the first season, Katara dons this hairstyle, which features her famous loopies!

SKILL LEVEL: Easy
TIME: 15 minutes

MATERIALS NEEDED:

Hair clips

1 small hair elastic

4 hair beads

2 small, clear hair elastics (optional)

1 large hair elastic

Topsy tail

Bobby pins

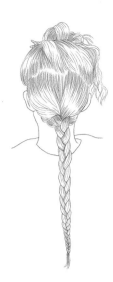

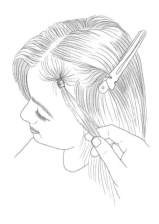

I. Horizontally divide the hair in half. Secure the top half on top of the head with a clip for now, then English-braid the bottom half to the ends and secure with a small hair elastic.

2. Take two small sections of hair at the forehead on either side of a center part. Place one bead on each of these sections, making sure the beads stay at the roots of the hair. If you're having trouble keeping the beads in place, tie small, clear hair elastics in the hair first, then slide the beads over them.

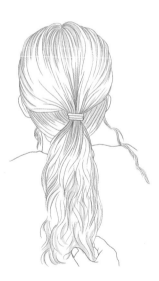

3. Tie the remaining hair into a ponytail, on top of where the braid starts, and secure with a large hair elastic.

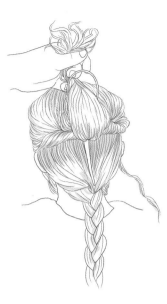

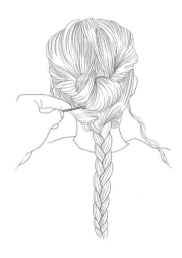

4. Using a topsy tail, flip the ponytail inside out. Keep doing this motion, and eventually the ponytail hair will all be wrapped around the hair elastic and form a bun. Pin the ends underneath the bun to hide them.

5. Drape the front hair sections back and pin the ends into the sides of the bun.

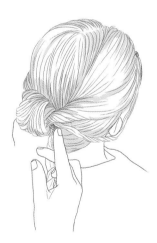

6. Pin two more beads into this bun where the front sections join it by placing each bead onto the crook of a bobby pin.

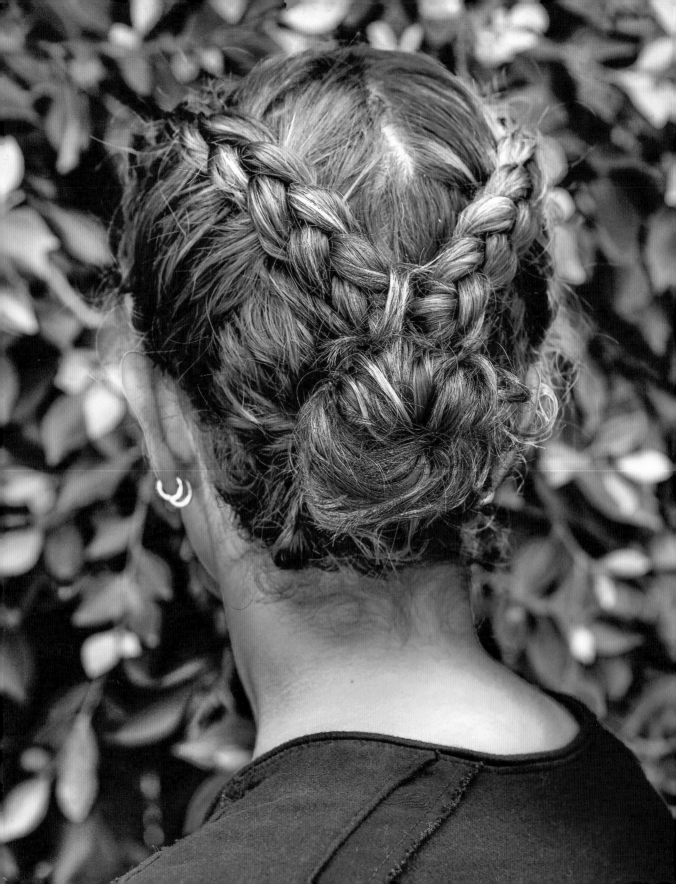

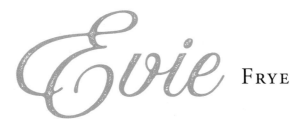

Evie F**RYE**

It's 1868 in the polluted city of London, and twin siblings Jacob and Evie Frye are recruited by the British Brotherhood of Assassins to defeat a powerful Templar boss named Starrick. Luckily Evie's stealth and smarts are a good complement to Jacob's combat prowess as they encounter Templars and gangsters who are hell-bent on thwarting their mission. Evie needs a clear view as she leaps from buildings and wrestles with evil henchmen, so this braided updo is a practical look that keeps hair neatly and stylishly away from the face.

SKILL LEVEL: Intermediate
TIME: 15 minutes

MATERIALS NEEDED:

2 small hair elastics
1 large hair elastic
Bobby pins

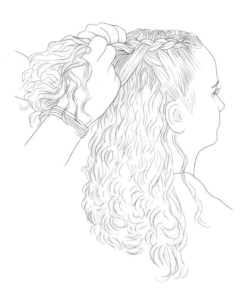

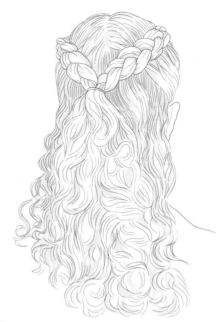

1. Make a slight side part. On one side of the head, make a Dutch braid, starting at the corner of the forehead and going backward. Stop adding in hair once you get past the ears, then English-braid the hair to the ends. Secure with a small hair elastic for now. Repeat this step on the other side of the head.

2. Join these Dutch braids together at the center of the back of the head with a large hair elastic. Undo the braiding below this elastic.

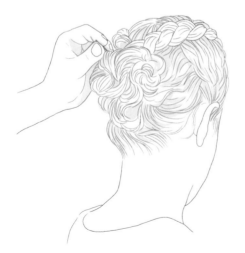

3. Gather up the remaining hair and twist it tightly. Coil this twist into a bun, making sure it covers the hair elastic holding the braids together. Pin this bun in place with bobby pins.

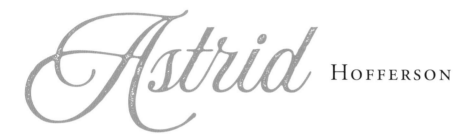 HOFFERSON

This teenaged Viking dragon rider is known for her axe-wielding skills and her fierce attitude. Now, with the help of her Black Nadder Stormfly, she must defend her village and save the dragons of the world from the ruthless dragon-hunter Drago Bludvist, who wants to control them all for his own ends. Why not do it in style?

SKILL LEVEL: Intermediate
TIME: 15 minutes

MATERIALS NEEDED:

1 small hair elastic
Leather headband
1 large hair elastic

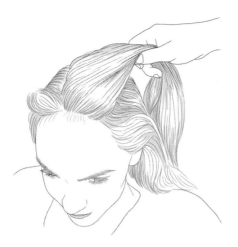

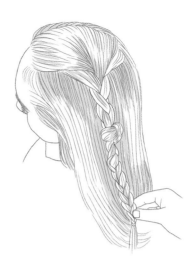

1. Make a deep side part. On the bigger side of the part, gather up a section of hair, leaving out any bangs.

2. Switch off between English-braiding and knot-braiding this section of hair—this means make an English braid for a little length of the strands, then tie a knot with one of the strands and start making an English braid again. Make another knot, and so on. Do this for the whole length of the section and secure it with the small hair elastic.

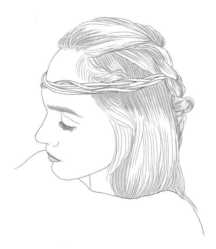

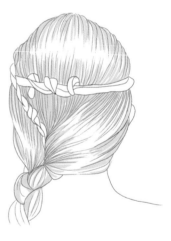

3. Tie the leather headband across the forehead, underneath the accent braid and over the rest of the hair.

4. Now gather the remaining hair to the side of the head, where the accent braid is, and switch off between English-braiding and knot-braiding this hair too. The accent braid should be incorporated into this braid as one of the strands. Secure the ends with the large hair elastic.

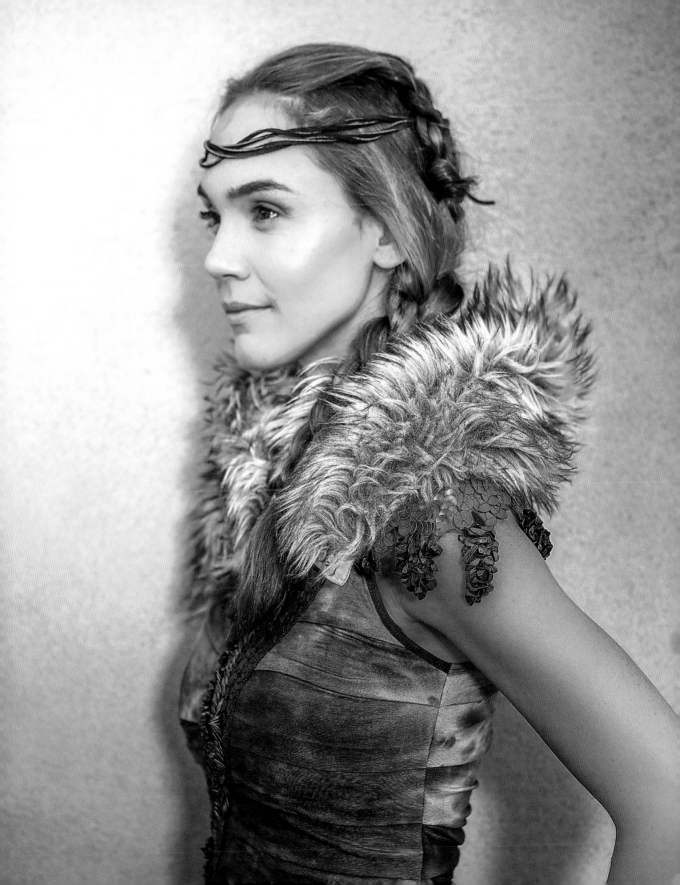

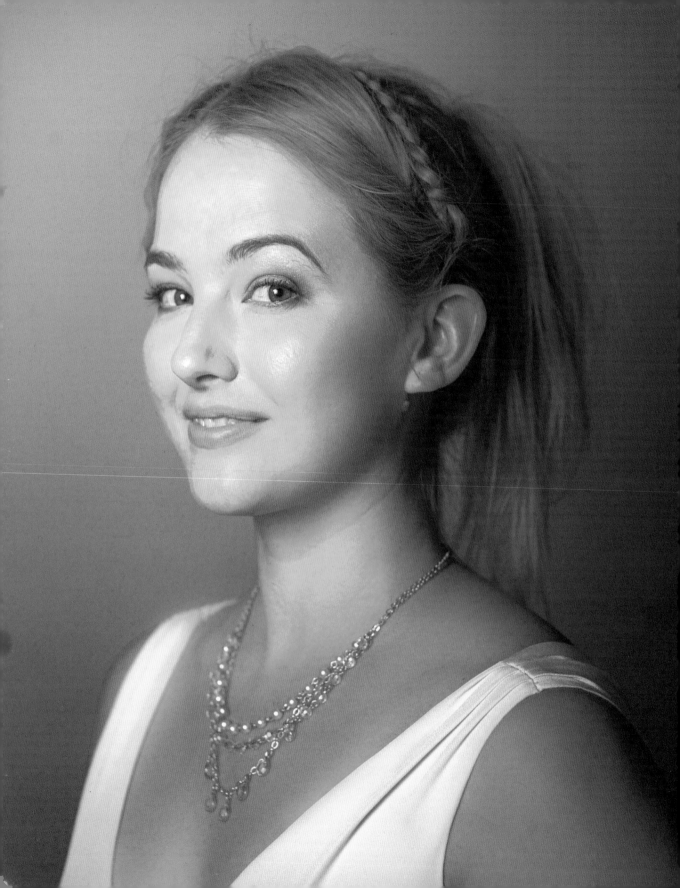

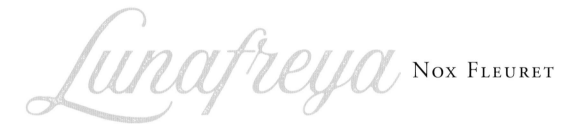 Nox Fleuret

Final Fantasy XV heroine Lunafreya is the former princess of Tenebrae and the youngest Oracle in history. Now it is up to her to stop the spread of the Starscourge plague from plunging the world of Eos into eternal darkness and being overrun by daemons. Will she succeed?

Most *Final Fantasy* characters have the typical spiky anime hair that doesn't really work for real-world styling, but Luna's braids and flipped ponytail are easy to recreate.

SKILL LEVEL: Intermediate
TIME: 15 minutes

MATERIALS NEEDED:

Hair clips

1 large hair elastic

Topsy tail (optional)

Bobby pins

1 small, clear hair elastic

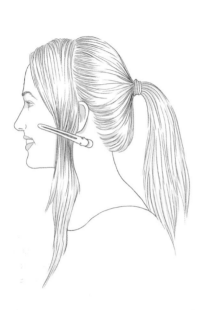

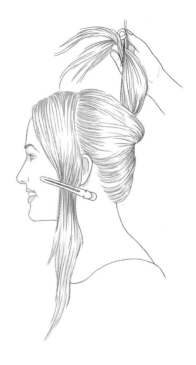

1. Make a center part. Leave out any bangs and part them on the side. On each side of the center part, gather a section of hair between the forehead hair and the ear and clip it out of the way. Tie the rest of hair back into a ponytail in the center of the back of the head, and secure it with a large hair elastic.

2. With a topsy tail or your fingers, flip this ponytail inside out so the tail sticks upward.

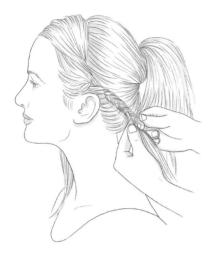 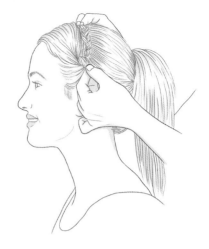

3. With one of the sections of hair clipped out of the way, twist it back a bit, then English-braid it to the ends and clip them for now. Repeat this step with the section of clipped hair on the other side of the head.

4. Pin these two braids over the top of the head with bobby pins. Then secure each of the braids with a small, clear hair elastic, positioning each elastic so that it is level with the twisted part of the other braid. If there is extra length to the tail of these braids, let it hang freely behind the ears.

{ DID YOU KNOW?

Hair is notoriously difficult to animate. In early animated movies, most hairstyles look like a solid blob of straight hair because of the challenge rendering millions of individual hairs. When computer-generated imagery (CGI) arrived, however, the video game Final Fantasy broke significant ground in animating hair where individual strands could move independently. Nowadays, computers are powerful enough to render images and movement patterns for hundreds of thousands of hairs at once. Moviemakers even run complex physics simulations in order to make animated curly hair look realistic.

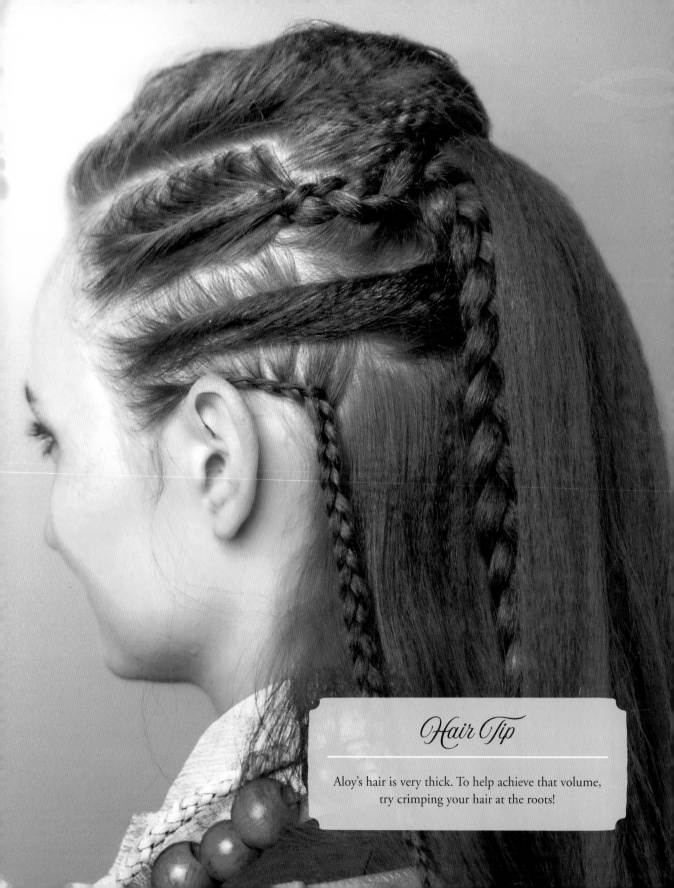

Hair Tip

Aloy's hair is very thick. To help achieve that volume, try crimping your hair at the roots!

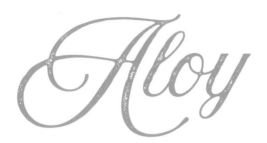

Aloy is the protagonist in the post-apocalyptic environment of *Horizon Zero Dawn*, which is overrun by animal-like robots that have been corrupted by a mysterious force. Cast out of the Nora tribe as a baby, Aloy later proves that she is a kickass warrior who can go head-to-head with any adversary and win, thanks in part to her superb archery skills and some "old-world" technology.

The hairstyles of the Nora tribe involve thick twists, dreads, and braids, which Aloy shows off through the entire game.

SKILL LEVEL: Advanced
TIME: 30 minutes

MATERIALS NEEDED:
9 small hair elastics
Hair clips
Crimping iron (optional)

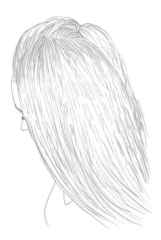

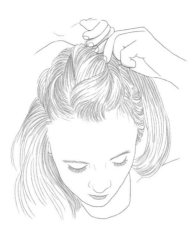

1. Section off one-third of the hair on top of the head, running from front to back. Start twisting this section, adding in more hair as you move backward. Secure with a small hair elastic at the crown.

2. Twist up another third of the hair on top of the head. Make sure to twist toward the middle of the head. Clip this twist in back for now. Twist up the last third of hair as well so that all the hair on top of the head is twisted.

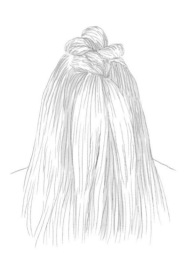

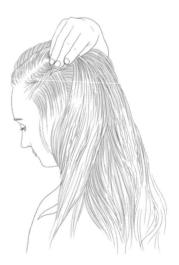

3. Cross the outer twists over the elastic holding the middle twist, then tie these twists together underneath the first elastic. Gently tug on little bits of the twists to fluff them out.

4. On both sides of the head, divide the hair in two horizontally. Twist the first half of the top section.

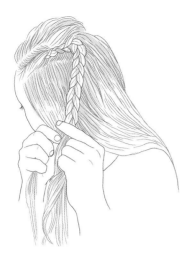

5. Halfway back, transition into making a Dutch lace braid and incorporate the rest of the hair in this section. Stop adding in hair when you reach the ponytail, and then finish the braid to the ends, securing with a small hair elastic. Repeat with the twist on the other side of the head.

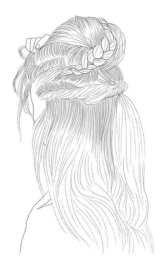

6. Make another twist on each side of the head with the bottom halves of side hair, leaving out a little bit of hair above the ears. Tie these twists together at the back of the head underneath the braids and the ponytail.

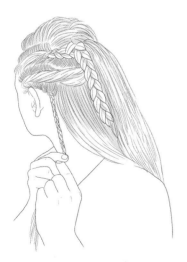

7. Make small Dutch lace braids with the remaining hair above the ears.

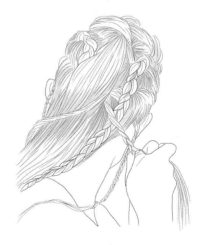

8. Finally, make two more English braids from the hair behind the head so that each one falls over each shoulder.

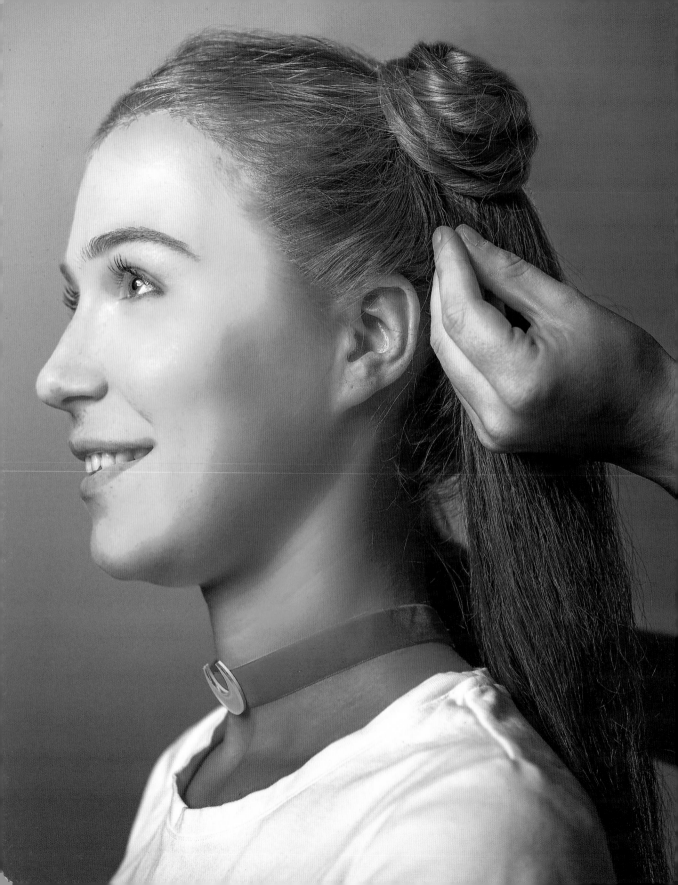

Acknowledgments

I would like to give a big thank you to everyone who made this book possible! Without you, there wouldn't even be the inkling of an idea for this project. First, a shout out to everyone at Quarto for inviting me to write this and for pulling this book together in a hurry, including the editorial staff (Melanie Madden, Jeannine Dillon, Erin Canning, Heather Rodino) and the design team (Merideth Harte, Melissa Gerber). Thank you to Fortuna Todisco for creating all the step-by-step illustrations, and Frank Hom for spending a full four days with me taking photographs of all the different hairstyles in this book.

A special shout out goes to to all the models who let me do their hair: Ashlyn Madden, Anna Smirnova, Dawn Desvigne, Andy Baptiste, Lucy Shen, Macrina Cooper-White, Maya Waeger, Kimi Beck, Kevin Burke, and Jess Shropshire. You guys were amazing. Also, special thanks to Kate Marley for the awesome makeup!

Last but not least, I would like to thank my Aunt Michelle, for teaching me to braid all those years ago; my hair mentors and good friends Siobhan Retsina and Heather Eberly, whose guidance helped me develop my styling enough to show it to you all; my parents for their unwavering support; and my boyfriend, Eli, for all his patience and love.

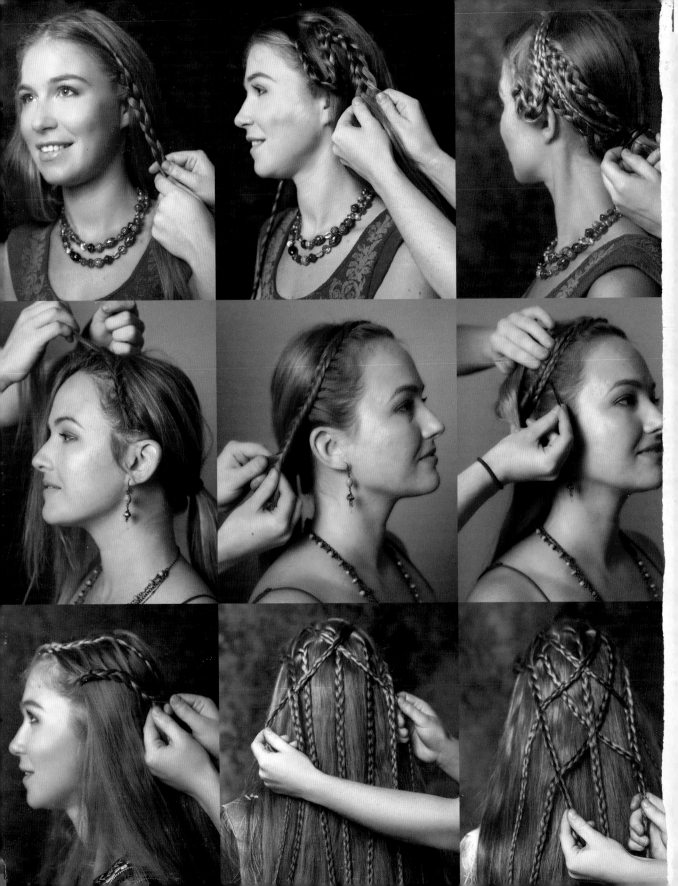